# RESTFUL NIGHTS: MEDITATION AND BREATHING TECHNIQUES FOR BETTER SLEEP

# TABLE OF CONTENT

# INTRODUCTION

Welcome to "Restful Nights: Meditation and Breathing Techniques for Better Sleep," a comprehensive guide designed to unlock the path to rejuvenating sleep and transform your well-being. In the hustle and bustle of our modern world, attaining quality sleep has become a challenge for many individuals in the prime years of adulthood, where the weight of work, family, and responsibilities can take a toll on restfulness. In this book, we delve deep into the significance of sleep for overall health, exploring the detrimental effects of poor sleep on daily life and productivity. Through the art of meditation and harnessing the power of breath, we offer practical tools to create a sleep-conducive environment and establish healthy sleep habits.

The journey to better sleep commences with a profound understanding of the science of sleep and our circadian rhythms. We will explore how these natural cycles regulate our sleep-wake patterns and delve into external factors, such as light and technology, that can significantly impact our sleep quality. Equipped with this knowledge, you can begin to establish effective routines to promote serene nights and invigorating days.

Meditation serves as a potent tool to quiet the mind, reduce stress, and is an essential element of our approach. Supported by scientific evidence that highlights meditation's positive effects on sleep quality, you'll be inspired to embrace these ancient practices. Alongside meditation, we'll explore the art of breathing and its profound connection to the nervous system. With a collection of simple yet powerful breathing techniques, you can effortlessly ease anxiety and create a sense of calm before bedtime.

Your sleep environment plays a pivotal role in your quest for better rest, and we provide valuable insights into optimizing your bedroom atmosphere. From minimizing noise and light disturbances to incorporating the benefits of aromatherapy and soothing sounds, we leave no stone unturned to ensure an oasis of tranquility where sleep can flourish.

In "Restful Nights: Meditation and Breathing Techniques for Blissful Sleep," we empower you to take full control of your sleep journey, offering a holistic approach that addresses not only the physical aspects of sleep but also the mental and emotional components. By wholeheartedly embracing the practices and techniques shared in this book, you'll embark on a transformative experience that culminates in a well-rested life filled with vitality and crystal-clear clarity. Say goodbye to restless nights, and get ready to embrace a new dawn of deeply restful, rejuvenating sleep.

# CHAPTER 1: UNDERSTANDING SLEEP AND ITS IMPORTANCE

Sleep is an indispensable aspect of human life, playing a vital role in our physical and mental well-being. It is during restful slumber that our bodies undergo essential restorative processes, allowing us to awaken refreshed and ready to embrace the day. In the first chapter, "Understanding Sleep and Its Importance," we delve into the significance of quality sleep and its profound impact on our overall health.

Quality sleep is not a mere luxury; it is a necessity for optimal functioning. As we explore the significance of sleep, we come to deeply appreciate its role in maintaining a balanced and vibrant life. From bolstering our immune system function to supporting cognitive processes and emotional well-being, sleep stands as a cornerstone of our vitality.

Unfortunately, in our fast-paced modern era, a restful night's sleep has become a challenging quest for many individuals, particularly those who face the weight of demanding responsibilities, be it work, family, or other obligations. We shed light on common sleep problems faced by those navigating the demands of today's world, emphasizing the importance of addressing these issues to enhance their daily lives.

The repercussions of poor sleep extend well beyond the night hours, impacting our productivity, focus, and overall mood throughout the day. By understanding the profound relationship between sleep and our daily functioning, we are inspired to prioritize and elevate our sleep habits to new heights.

As we embark on this transformative journey called "Restful Nights," we warmly invite you to explore the science of sleep, recognizing its immeasurable value. Through proactive and insightful steps, we shall uncover the mysteries of sleep, peering into the influence of various factors on our sleep patterns. Ultimately, we shall equip you with a treasure trove of meditation and breathing techniques, opening the door to nights that are both deeply restful and profoundly rejuvenating.

## The Significance Of Quality Sleep For Physical And Mental Well-Being

Quality sleep is not merely a luxury but a fundamental pillar of overall physical and mental well-being. The significance of sleep cannot be overstated, as it plays a vital role in supporting and maintaining our health on multiple levels.

Physically, sleep is a restorative process that allows our bodies to heal and repair. During sleep, our tissues and muscles undergo repair and growth, while our immune system strengthens its defenses against illnesses and infections. Quality sleep is essential for cardiovascular health, as it helps regulate blood pressure and reduce the risk of heart-related conditions.

Mentally, sleep is equally crucial for cognitive function and emotional well-being. While we sleep, our brains consolidate memories, process information, and enhance learning and problem-solving abilities. Adequate sleep is closely linked to improved focus, concentration, and creativity during waking hours. On the emotional front, getting enough rest can regulate mood and help manage stress, anxiety, and depression.

Furthermore, quality sleep is intertwined with our hormonal balance. Sleep influences the production of hormones like cortisol, which affects stress levels, and hormones that regulate hunger and appetite. Poor sleep patterns can disrupt these hormonal balances, potentially leading to weight gain and other health issues.

The absence of quality sleep can lead to a myriad of adverse effects on our physical and mental health. Chronic sleep deprivation has been associated with a higher risk of developing chronic conditions such as obesity, diabetes, and cardiovascular diseases. It can also impair our immune system, leaving us more vulnerable to infections and illnesses.

Moreover, inadequate sleep impacts our cognitive abilities,

memory retention, and decision-making skills. It can lead to decreased productivity, difficulty in learning, and reduced overall mental sharpness. Emotionally, lack of sleep is linked to irritability, mood swings, and an increased risk of anxiety and depression.

In "Restful Nights," we aim to emphasize the immense value of quality sleep for both physical and mental well-being. By understanding the significance of sleep, we can take proactive steps to prioritize our rest and incorporate effective techniques, such as meditation and breathing exercises, to achieve better sleep and enjoy the myriad benefits it brings to our daily lives.

## Common Sleep Problems Faced By Individuals Balancing Work, Family, and Life Demands

Individuals balancing work, family, and various life demands often face a range of sleep problems that can disrupt their rest and impact their overall well-being. While sleep issues can vary from person to person, several common sleep problems are frequently experienced within this phase of life:

- **Insomnia:** Insomnia is a prevalent sleep disorder characterized by difficulty falling asleep, staying asleep, or waking up too early and not being able to return to sleep. The demands and stress of daily life can contribute to insomnia.

- **Sleep Apnea:** Sleep apnea is a sleep disorder where breathing repeatedly stops and starts during sleep. Factors such as weight gain and changes in muscle tone can be particularly relevant during this phase of life.

- **Restless Legs Syndrome (RLS):** RLS is a condition characterized by an irresistible urge to move the legs, usually due to discomfort or unpleasant sensations. It can disrupt sleep and lead to frequent awakenings.

- **Shift Work Sleep Disorder:** Many individuals in this age range may work irregular or night shifts, leading to misalignment of their circadian rhythms and difficulty sleeping during unconventional hours.

- **Stress and Anxiety:** This phase of life can be filled with significant life changes, career challenges, and family responsibilities, leading to increased stress and anxiety levels that can impact sleep quality.

- **Narcolepsy:** While less common, narcolepsy can manifest in this age group, causing excessive daytime sleepiness, sudden loss of muscle control (cataplexy), and disrupted nighttime sleep.

- **Technology and Screen Time:** Excessive use of electronic devices and screen time before bedtime can lead to sleep problems due to the disruption of natural sleep-wake cycles caused by blue light exposure.

- **Alcohol and Caffeine:** Consuming alcohol and caffeine close to bedtime can interfere with sleep quality and contribute to sleep disturbances.

- **Environmental Factors:** Noise, light pollution, uncomfortable bedroom temperatures, and other environmental factors can disrupt sleep during this dynamic phase of life.

- **Restless Sleep Patterns:** Some individuals may experience fragmented or restless sleep due to lifestyle factors, inconsistent sleep schedules, or unidentified underlying sleep disorders.

Addressing these sleep problems is essential to improve sleep quality and overall well-being. In "Restful Nights," we explore effective strategies, meditation, and breathing techniques that can help individuals balancing work, family, and life demands overcome these sleep challenges and enjoy more restful nights for a healthier and more fulfilling life.

## *The Negative Effects Of Poor Sleep On Daily Life And Productivity*

The negative effects of poor sleep on daily life and productivity are far-reaching and can have a significant impact on various aspects of our physical, mental, and emotional well-being. When we consistently fail to get adequate and restful sleep, several detrimental consequences emerge:

- **Cognitive Impairment:** Sleep is essential for cognitive functions such as attention, concentration, and memory. Poor sleep can lead to reduced focus, impaired decision-making, and difficulty retaining information, affecting overall cognitive performance.

- **Reduced Productivity:** Fatigue and lack of energy resulting from poor sleep can lead to decreased productivity and efficiency in both professional and personal tasks. Individuals may find it challenging to complete tasks on time, leading to increased stress and anxiety.

- **Mood Disturbances:** Insufficient sleep is closely linked to mood swings, irritability, and heightened emotional reactivity. It can exacerbate feelings of stress, anxiety, and depression, impacting interpersonal relationships and overall emotional well-being.

- **Weakened Immune System:** Sleep plays a critical role in supporting the immune system. Chronic sleep deprivation weakens the immune response, making individuals more susceptible to infections and illnesses.

- **Impaired Physical Health:** Poor sleep is associated with an increased risk of various health issues, including obesity, diabetes, cardiovascular diseases, and hypertension. It can disrupt the body's hormonal balance, leading to potential long-term health consequences.

- **Risk of Accidents:** Fatigue resulting from inadequate sleep can impair motor skills and reaction times, increasing the risk of accidents at home, work, or while driving.

- **Lack of Energy and Motivation:** A consistent lack of quality sleep can lead to persistent feelings of tiredness and low energy, making it challenging to engage in physical activities or pursue personal interests.

- **Difficulty Coping with Stress:** Quality sleep is essential for stress management. Poor sleep can intensify the body's stress response, making it harder to cope with daily challenges and leading to a cycle of increased stress and worsened sleep.

- **Impaired Creativity and Innovation:** A well-rested mind is more capable of creative thinking and problem-solving. In contrast, poor sleep can hinder creativity and innovative thinking, limiting potential breakthroughs in various aspects of life.

- **Relationship Strain:** Sleep disturbances can affect relationships with partners, family members, and friends. Irritability and mood swings may lead to conflicts and strained interpersonal dynamics.

Addressing and improving sleep quality is crucial for mitigating these negative effects. In "Restful Nights," we equip individuals with effective meditation and breathing techniques, as well as other valuable strategies, to promote better sleep habits and break free from the cycle of poor sleep, leading to enhanced daily life and increased productivity.

# CHAPTER 2: THE SCIENCE OF SLEEP AND CIRCADIAN RHYTHMS

The science of sleep and circadian rhythms forms the foundation for understanding the natural cycles that regulate our sleep-wake patterns and influence our overall well-being. These biological processes are governed by intricate systems within our bodies, and a deeper understanding of them can empower us to optimize our sleep and improve our quality of life.

- **Circadian Rhythms:** At the core of the science of sleep lies the concept of circadian rhythms. These are 24-hour internal cycles that regulate various physiological and behavioral processes, including our sleep-wake cycles. The suprachiasmatic nucleus (SCN), a tiny region in the brain's hypothalamus, serves as the body's internal clock, coordinating these rhythms with external cues such as light and darkness.

The primary external factor that influences our circadian rhythms is the natural light-dark cycle. When light enters our eyes, it signals the SCN to suppress the production of the sleep-inducing hormone melatonin, promoting wakefulness. As darkness sets in, melatonin levels rise, signaling the body to prepare for sleep. Disruptions to this light-dark cycle, such as shift work or excessive exposure to artificial light during nighttime, can lead to circadian misalignment and sleep problems.

- **The Sleep-Wake Cycle:** The sleep-wake cycle is an essential component of circadian rhythms. Throughout the day, we experience fluctuations in alertness and sleepiness, with the drive to sleep peaking at night and alertness peaking during the day. This pattern is regulated by the interaction between the SCN, melatonin levels, and other neurotransmitters and hormones in the brain.


- **Sleep Stages:** During sleep, our bodies undergo distinct stages that make up a sleep cycle. These stages include non-rapid eye movement (NREM) sleep, which is divided into three stages (N1, N2, and N3), and rapid eye movement (REM) sleep. Each stage plays a unique role in the restorative and cognitive processes of sleep.

  NREM sleep helps restore the body, promoting physical recovery and rejuvenation. During REM sleep, our brains are highly active, facilitating memory consolidation, emotional processing, and dreaming. Throughout the night, we cycle through these stages multiple times, with REM sleep becoming more prominent as the night progresses.


- **Factors Impacting Sleep:** In addition to circadian rhythms, various factors can influence our sleep patterns. These include lifestyle choices, stress levels, dietary habits, and exposure to electronic devices before bedtime. Understanding how these factors interact with our circadian rhythms can help us make informed decisions to improve our sleep hygiene and overall sleep quality.


In "Restful Nights," we explore the delicate science of sleep and circadian rhythms, empowering individuals to align their habits and routines with these natural cycles. By establishing healthy sleep practices that honor the body's internal clock, we can optimize our sleep, enhance daytime alertness, and pave the way for more restful, rejuvenating nights.

## *Explaining The Circadian Rhythm*
## *And Its Role In Sleep-Wake Cycles*

The circadian rhythm is an essential biological process that regulates various physiological and behavioral functions in living organisms, including humans. Derived from the Latin words "circa" (around) and "diem" (day), circadian rhythms are approximately 24-hour cycles that synchronize an organism's internal processes with the external environment, primarily the light-dark cycle of day and night.

In humans, the master regulator of the circadian rhythm is a tiny region in the brain's hypothalamus known as the suprachiasmatic nucleus (SCN). The SCN serves as the body's internal clock and is responsible for orchestrating the timing of various bodily functions, including the sleep-wake cycle, hormone secretion, body temperature, and metabolism.

The primary external cue that synchronizes our internal clock with the external environment is light. Photoreceptors in the retina of our eyes detect light, and this information is transmitted to the SCN, which then signals the pineal gland to regulate the production of the hormone melatonin.

Melatonin, often referred to as the "sleep hormone," plays a crucial role in the sleep-wake cycle. Its secretion is suppressed by light and increases in response to darkness. As daylight diminishes in the evening, the rise in melatonin levels signals to the body that it is time to prepare for sleep. Conversely, when we are exposed to natural light in the morning, melatonin production decreases, signaling wakefulness and alertness.

Throughout the night, the interaction between the SCN and melatonin production drives the sleep-wake cycle. As melatonin levels rise, we experience increasing drowsiness and transition into sleep. During the night, we go through cycles of non-rapid eye movement (NREM) sleep, which consists of three stages (N1, N2, and N3), and rapid eye movement (REM) sleep.

NREM sleep is responsible for physical restoration and recovery, promoting bodily rest and repairing tissues. REM sleep, on the other hand, is associated with heightened brain activity, and it is crucial for cognitive functions such as memory consolidation and emotional processing. As the night progresses, REM sleep becomes more prominent, and our sleep cycles alternate between NREM and REM sleep several times.

Disruptions to the circadian rhythm, such as shift work, jet lag, or irregular sleep schedules, can lead to circadian misalignment. When our internal clock is out of sync with the external environment, we may experience difficulties falling asleep or staying awake at desired times, leading to sleep disturbances and reduced overall sleep quality.

Understanding the role of the circadian rhythm in the sleep-wake cycle is vital for optimizing our sleep habits and promoting restful nights. By aligning our daily routines with our natural circadian rhythms, we can enhance the synchronization between our internal clock and the external environment, leading to improved sleep quality and overall well-being.

## *How External Factors Like Light And Technology Impact Sleep Patterns*

External factors like light and technology can significantly impact sleep patterns and overall sleep quality. Here's how:

- **Light:**

  - **Circadian Rhythm:** The circadian rhythm is our internal biological clock that regulates the sleep-wake cycle. Light exposure, especially natural light during the day and darkness at night, plays a crucial role in synchronizing this rhythm. Exposure to natural light during the day helps regulate the circadian rhythm and promotes better sleep at night.

  - **Melatonin Production:** Melatonin is a hormone that helps control sleep-wake cycles. Light, especially blue light emitted by electronic devices (phones, tablets, computers), can suppress melatonin production. Evening exposure to bright screens can disrupt the body's ability to prepare for sleep, leading to difficulties falling asleep and reduced sleep duration.

  - **Sleep Environment:** Bright artificial light in the bedroom, such as streetlights or electronics with LED displays, can interfere with sleep quality. Using blackout curtains and minimizing light exposure during the night can improve sleep.

- **Technology:**

  - **Screen Time:** As mentioned earlier, electronic devices emit blue light that can interfere with melatonin production. Additionally, engaging in stimulating activities like playing video games, watching action-packed movies, or using social media can make it harder for individuals to wind down before bedtime.

- **Sleep Disturbances:** Alerts, notifications, and the temptation to check devices during the night can lead to sleep disruptions. Vibrations, sounds, or even the anticipation of messages can disturb sleep and reduce sleep continuity.

- **Sleep Disorders:** Excessive use of technology can lead to sleep disorders like insomnia or sleep deprivation due to extended screen time, irregular sleep schedules, and reduced exposure to natural light during the day.

To mitigate the impact of light and technology on sleep patterns:

- **Practice good sleep hygiene:** Establish a regular sleep schedule, create a relaxing bedtime routine, and avoid stimulating activities before bed.

- **Limit screen time before bedtime:** Avoid using electronic devices at least an hour before sleep. Consider using "night mode" settings on devices or installing blue light filters.

- **Control bedroom lighting:** Use blackout curtains or eye masks to minimize light exposure during sleep.

- **Prioritize natural light exposure:** Spend time outdoors during the day, especially in the morning, to regulate the circadian rhythm.

- **Establish a technology-free bedroom:** Keep electronic devices out of the bedroom to minimize distractions and sleep disturbances.

By being mindful of these external factors and making positive changes to sleep habits, individuals can improve their sleep patterns and overall sleep quality.

## *Establishing Healthy Sleep Habits And Routines For Better Rest*

Establishing healthy sleep habits and routines is essential for getting better rest and improving overall sleep quality. Here are some tips to help you achieve a good night's sleep:

- **Maintain a Consistent Sleep Schedule:** Go to bed and wake up at the same time every day, even on weekends. This helps regulate your body's internal clock and improves the quality of your sleep.

- **Create a Relaxing Bedtime Routine:** Develop a calming pre-sleep routine to signal your body that it's time to wind down. This can include activities such as reading a book, taking a warm bath, practicing relaxation techniques, or gentle stretching.

- **Limit Screen Time Before Bed:** Avoid using electronic devices with screens (e.g., smartphones, computers, and TVs) at least an hour before bedtime. The blue light emitted by these devices can disrupt the production of the sleep hormone melatonin, making it harder to fall asleep.

- **Create a Sleep-Friendly Environment:** Make your bedroom conducive to sleep by keeping it dark, quiet, and cool. Use blackout curtains or an eye mask to block out light, and consider using earplugs or white noise machines to mask any disruptive sounds.

- **Be Mindful of What You Consume:** Avoid heavy meals, caffeine, nicotine, and alcohol close to bedtime. These substances can interfere with your ability to fall asleep and stay asleep.

- **Stay Active During the Day:** Regular physical activity can improve sleep quality, but try to avoid vigorous exercise close to bedtime, as it may make it harder to fall asleep.

- **Limit Naps:** While short daytime naps can be refreshing, avoid long or late-afternoon naps, as they may interfere with your ability to sleep at night.

- **Manage Stress:** Practice stress-reduction techniques such as meditation, deep breathing exercises, or journaling to help calm your mind before bedtime.

- **Get Exposure to Natural Light:** Spend time outdoors during the day, especially in the morning. Exposure to natural light helps regulate your circadian rhythm and promotes better sleep at night.

- **Limit Alcohol and Caffeine:** While alcohol may initially make you feel drowsy, it can disrupt sleep patterns and lead to poorer sleep quality. Similarly, caffeine can interfere with falling asleep and may reduce sleep duration if consumed too close to bedtime.

- **Don't Force Sleep:** If you can't fall asleep within 20-30 minutes of going to bed, get up and do something relaxing in dim light until you feel sleepy.

- **Keep a Sleep Diary:** Tracking your sleep patterns and habits can help identify potential issues and guide you in making improvements.

Remember that building healthy sleep habits may take time, so be patient with yourself as you make these changes. By adopting these habits and sticking to a consistent sleep routine, you can improve the quality and quantity of your rest, leading to better overall well-being. If sleep problems persist despite making these changes, consider seeking advice from a healthcare professional or sleep specialist.

# CHAPTER 3: MEDITATION AND ITS IMPACT ON SLEEP

Meditation can have a positive impact on sleep and can help improve sleep quality in various ways. Here's how meditation can influence sleep:

- **Reduces Stress and Anxiety:** One of the primary benefits of meditation is its ability to reduce stress and anxiety. When practiced regularly, meditation can help calm the mind, promote relaxation, and reduce the physiological response to stress. Lowering stress levels can make it easier to fall asleep and improve overall sleep quality.

- **Promotes Mindfulness and Awareness:** Meditation cultivates mindfulness, which involves being fully present and aware of the present moment without judgment. By practicing mindfulness, individuals can let go of ruminating thoughts that may keep them awake at night, leading to better sleep.

- **Enhances Sleep Quality:** Meditation has been shown to increase the production of melatonin, the hormone responsible for regulating sleep-wake cycles. As a result, improved melatonin levels can lead to more restful and deeper sleep.

- **Helps with Insomnia:** Insomnia is often associated with racing thoughts and an inability to relax. Meditation can address these issues by calming the mind and reducing the mental chatter that interferes with falling asleep. The practice can also help establish a bedtime routine, making it easier for individuals with insomnia to signal their bodies that it's time to sleep.

- **Improves Sleep Duration:** Regular meditation has been linked to increased total sleep time. By helping individuals fall asleep faster and experience fewer nighttime awakenings, meditation can lead to longer and more restorative sleep.

- **Reduces Sleep Disturbances:** Meditation can decrease the occurrence of sleep disturbances like nightmares and night terrors. It creates a more peaceful and stable mental state that can prevent disruptive sleep episodes.

- **Boosts Sleep Satisfaction:** Meditators often report feeling more satisfied with their sleep patterns and overall sleep quality. This increased satisfaction may be due to the calming and centering effects of meditation, which can carry over into the sleep experience.

- **May Help with Sleep Disorders:** While not a cure, meditation can be used as an adjunctive therapy to manage certain sleep disorders like insomnia, sleep apnea, and restless legs syndrome. It complements other treatment strategies by promoting relaxation and reducing sleep-related anxiety.

It's important to note that the benefits of meditation on sleep may vary from person to person, and some individuals may experience improvements more quickly than others. Consistency and patience are essential when integrating meditation into a sleep improvement plan. Also, meditation is generally considered safe for most people, but if you have any medical or psychological conditions, it's a good idea to consult with a healthcare professional before starting a meditation practice or using it as a primary treatment for sleep issues.

## *Introduction To Meditation As A Tool To Calm The Mind And Reduce Stress*

In today's fast-paced and hectic world, stress and anxiety have become common challenges that affect our mental and physical well-being. Fortunately, meditation offers a simple and effective solution to help calm the mind and reduce stress. Meditation is an ancient practice that has been used for thousands of years to promote relaxation, inner peace, and overall well-being.

**What is Meditation?** Meditation is a practice that involves training the mind to focus and redirect thoughts, allowing individuals to attain a heightened state of awareness and deep relaxation. It often involves focusing attention on a specific object, thought, or activity, or simply being mindful of the present moment without judgment.

**How Does Meditation Work?** During meditation, practitioners learn to observe their thoughts without becoming attached to them. This process helps to create a sense of detachment from the constant stream of thoughts and worries that may contribute to stress. By redirecting the focus inward, individuals can experience a sense of calm and gain clarity, reducing the impact of external stressors.

**Benefits of Meditation for Stress Reduction:**

- **Stress Reduction:** Meditation activates the body's relaxation response, which helps reduce stress hormones like cortisol and adrenaline. Regular practice can lead to a decreased overall stress level.

- **Improved Emotional Well-being:** Meditation can increase positive emotions, such as joy and compassion while reducing negative emotions like anxiety and depression.

- **Enhanced Self-awareness:** Through meditation, individuals develop a deeper understanding of their thoughts and emotions, which can lead to better self-regulation and emotional resilience.

- **Better Concentration and Focus:** Meditation trains the mind to concentrate on the present moment, which can improve focus and mental clarity.

- **Lower Blood Pressure:** Meditation has been associated with reduced blood pressure levels, which is beneficial for cardiovascular health.

- **Quality Sleep:** As mentioned earlier, meditation can improve sleep quality by calming the mind and reducing sleep disturbances related to stress and anxiety.

**Getting Started with Meditation:**

- **Choose a Comfortable Environment:** Find a quiet and peaceful space where you can sit or lie down comfortably without distractions.

- **Pick a Meditation Technique:** There are various meditation techniques to choose from, such as mindfulness meditation, loving-kindness meditation, and guided meditation. Experiment with different methods to find the one that resonates with you.

- **Start with Short Sessions:** Beginners can start with just a few minutes of meditation each day and gradually increase the duration as they become more comfortable with the practice.

- **Focus on Your Breath:** One of the simplest ways to begin is by focusing on your breath. Pay attention to the sensation of your breath as it goes in and out.

- **Be Gentle with Yourself:** It's natural for the mind to wander during meditation. When distractions arise, gently bring your focus back to your chosen point of meditation without self-judgment.

- **Practice Regularly:** Consistency is key. Aim to meditate daily, even if it's only for a short time. The benefits of meditation often become more apparent with regular practice.

Remember that meditation is a skill that improves over time, and the benefits may not be immediately noticeable. With patience and persistence, meditation can become a valuable tool for calming the mind, reducing stress, and enhancing overall well-being.

## *Scientific Evidence Supporting Meditation's Positive Effects On Sleep Quality*

Over the past few decades, a growing body of scientific research has explored the effects of meditation on sleep quality. Numerous studies have found evidence supporting the positive impact of meditation on various aspects of sleep. Here are some key findings from scientific research:

- **Reduced Insomnia Symptoms:** Several studies have shown that regular meditation can help reduce symptoms of insomnia, including difficulties falling asleep, staying asleep, and experiencing non-restorative sleep. Meditation techniques that promote relaxation and reduce arousal have been particularly effective in improving insomnia symptoms.

- **Improved Sleep Duration:** Research suggests that individuals who practice meditation regularly tend to have longer total sleep durations compared to those who do not meditate. Longer sleep duration is associated with better overall sleep quality and improved daytime functioning.

- **Enhanced Sleep Quality:** Meditation has been found to improve subjective sleep quality, as reported by individuals who practice meditation regularly. Meditators often report feeling more refreshed and rested upon waking, indicating better sleep quality.

- **Decreased Sleep Latency:** Sleep latency refers to the time it takes to fall asleep after getting into bed. Studies have shown that meditation can reduce sleep latency, helping individuals fall asleep more quickly.

- **Reduction in Sleep Disturbances:** Meditation has been associated with a decrease in sleep disturbances, such as waking up during the night or experiencing nightmares. Meditators often report fewer disruptions in their sleep patterns.

- **Impact on Sleep Architecture:** Some studies have explored the effects of meditation on sleep architecture, which refers to the various stages of sleep (e.g., REM sleep, deep sleep). While findings are mixed, there is evidence to suggest that meditation can influence sleep architecture positively.

- **Decreased Daytime Sleepiness:** Meditation has been linked to reduced daytime sleepiness and improved alertness during the day. By promoting better sleep at night, meditation can lead to increased daytime vitality.

- **Reduction in Sleep Medication Use:** Research has indicated that regular meditation practice can lead to a decrease in the use of sleep medications, as individuals experience improved sleep without relying on pharmaceutical aids.

It's important to note that individual responses to meditation may vary, and some studies have reported mixed results. Additionally, the specific meditation techniques used in research studies can influence the outcomes. However, overall, the evidence suggests that meditation can be a valuable tool for enhancing sleep quality and addressing sleep-related issues.

The mechanisms through which meditation positively affects sleep are still being explored, but it is believed that the relaxation response and stress reduction associated with meditation play a significant role. Meditation helps reduce sympathetic nervous system activity (associated with the fight-or-flight response) and enhances parasympathetic nervous system activity (associated with relaxation). These physiological changes contribute to improved sleep patterns and overall sleep quality.

As with any intervention, individual experiences may differ, and it's important to remember that meditation is not a replacement for medical advice or treatment for sleep disorders. If you have chronic sleep issues or concerns about your sleep quality, it's best to consult with a healthcare professional or sleep specialist for personalized guidance.

## Simple Meditation Techniques Suitable For Beginners

For beginners, it's best to start with simple meditation techniques that are easy to practice and don't require extensive experience or training. Here are some beginner-friendly meditation techniques to get you started:

- **Mindfulness Meditation:**
    a. Find a quiet and comfortable place to sit or lie down.
    b. Close your eyes or softly gaze at a fixed point.
    c. Focus your attention on your breath. Observe the sensation of your breath as you inhale and exhale.
    d. When your mind wanders (which is normal), gently bring your focus back to your breath without judgment.
- **Body Scan Meditation:**
    a. Lie down on your back or sit in a comfortable position with your eyes closed.
    b. Take a few deep breaths to relax your body and mind.
    c. Slowly direct your attention to each part of your body, starting from your toes and moving upward. Notice any sensations or tension in each area.
    d. As you focus on each body part, consciously relax and release any tension you feel.
- **Loving-Kindness Meditation (Metta Meditation):**
    a. Find a quiet place to sit comfortably.
    b. Close your eyes and take a few deep breaths to relax.
    c. Generate feelings of kindness and compassion toward yourself. Silently repeat phrases like

"May I be happy, may I be healthy, may I be safe."

    d. Extend these feelings of loving-kindness to others, starting with someone you care about, then to neutral people, and eventually even to those you may have difficulties with.

- **Guided Meditation:**
  a. Use pre-recorded guided meditation sessions. Many meditation apps and online resources offer guided meditations for various purposes, such as relaxation, stress reduction, and better sleep.
  b. Follow the instructions provided by the meditation guide, allowing them to lead you through the practice.

- **Breathing Meditation (Counting Breath):**
  a. Find a quiet place to sit comfortably.
  b. Close your eyes and take a few deep breaths to center yourself.
  c. As you breathe, count each breath cycle. For example, inhale deeply, and as you exhale, count "one." Inhale again, and as you exhale, count "two." Continue this pattern up to a count of ten, then start again from one.
  d. If your mind wanders, gently bring your focus back to counting your breaths.

- **Walking Meditation:**
  a. Find a quiet and safe place to walk, either indoors or outdoors.
  b. Walk at a comfortable pace, focusing your attention on each step you take.
  c. Feel the sensation of your feet touching the ground, the movement of your body, and the rhythm of your breath.
  d. If your mind drifts away, gently redirect your attention to the act of walking.

Remember that meditation is a skill that develops over time, so be patient with yourself and avoid self-judgment. Start with short sessions and gradually increase the duration as you become more comfortable. Consistency is more important than the length of each session, so try to incorporate meditation into your daily routine. As you continue to practice, you may find that meditation becomes a valuable tool for calming the mind, reducing stress, and enhancing your overall well-being.

# CHAPTER 4: BREATHING TECHNIQUES FOR RELAXATION

Breathing techniques can be incredibly effective for promoting relaxation and reducing stress. These techniques are simple, can be practiced almost anywhere, and are a great way to quickly calm the mind and body. Here are some popular breathing techniques for relaxation:

- **Deep Belly Breathing (Diaphragmatic Breathing):**
    a. Find a comfortable seated position or lie down on your back.

    b. Place one hand on your chest and the other on your abdomen.

    c. Inhale deeply through your nose, allowing your abdomen to rise as you fill your lungs with air. Make sure your chest stays relatively still.

    d. Exhale slowly and completely through your mouth, feeling your abdomen fall as you release the air.

    e. Focus on the sensation of your breath, and continue this deep belly breathing for a few minutes.

- **4-7-8 Breathing:**
    a. Sit in a comfortable position with your back straight.

    b. Inhale deeply through your nose to a count of 4.

    c. Hold your breath for a count of 7.

    d. Exhale slowly and completely through your mouth to a count of 8.

    e. Repeat this cycle for a few rounds, gradually increasing the duration if you feel comfortable.

- **Box Breathing (Square Breathing):**
    a. Sit or lie down in a relaxed position.

    b. Inhale deeply through your nose to a count of 4.

    c. Hold your breath for a count of 4.

    d. Exhale slowly and completely through your nose to a count of 4.

    e. Pause and hold your breath for another count of 4.

    f. Repeat this cycle for a few rounds, maintaining a steady and even rhythm.

- **Alternate Nostril Breathing (Nadi Shodhana):**
    a. Sit comfortably with your spine straight.

    b. Close your right nostril with your right thumb and inhale deeply through your left nostril.

    c. Close your left nostril with your right ring finger, release your right nostril, and exhale through the right nostril.

    d. Inhale deeply through your right nostril.

    e. Close your right nostril again, release your left nostril, and exhale through the left nostril.

    f. This completes one cycle. Continue the pattern for a few rounds, focusing on the smooth and controlled breath.

- **Humming Bee Breath (Bhramari Pranayama):**
  a. Find a comfortable seated position with your eyes closed.

  b. Place your thumbs on your ears and your index fingers over your closed eyes.

  c. Inhale deeply through your nose.

  d. As you exhale, make a soft humming sound like a bee, allowing the vibrations to resonate in your head.

  e. Repeat this process for a few rounds, focusing on the calming effect of the humming sound.

These breathing techniques can be practiced individually or combined with other relaxation techniques, such as meditation or progressive muscle relaxation. The key is to make breathing exercises a regular part of your routine, especially during moments of stress or when you need to relax and unwind. Over time, these techniques can help you build resilience to stress and promote a sense of calm and well-being in your daily life.

## *The Connection Between Breath And The Nervous System*

The connection between breath and the nervous system is profound and plays a crucial role in regulating our physiological and psychological states. The autonomic nervous system (ANS) is the part of the nervous system responsible for controlling involuntary bodily functions, including heart rate, digestion, respiratory rate, and more. It consists of two main branches: the sympathetic nervous system (SNS) and the parasympathetic nervous system (PNS).

- **Sympathetic Nervous System (SNS):**
    a. Also known as the "fight or flight" response, the SNS is activated in response to stress, danger, or perceived threats. When triggered, it prepares the body for action by increasing heart rate, constricting blood vessels, and releasing stress hormones like cortisol and adrenaline.

    b. Rapid and shallow breathing is a characteristic of SNS activation. This type of breathing is useful during emergencies or situations that require quick action.

- **Parasympathetic Nervous System (PNS):**
    a. The PNS is often referred to as the "rest and digest" response. It counteracts the effects of the SNS, promoting relaxation, recovery, and the conservation of energy.

    b. Slow and deep breathing is associated with PNS activation. This type of breathing helps induce a state of relaxation and calm.

**The Breath's Influence on the Nervous System:** The way we breathe directly influences the balance between the sympathetic and parasympathetic nervous systems, which, in turn, affects our overall well-being. Different breathing patterns can shift the body from a stressed, fight-or-flight mode to a relaxed, rest-and-digest state.

- **Stress Reduction:** Slow, deep, and controlled breathing activates the PNS, leading to reduced heart rate, lower blood pressure, and a decrease in stress hormone levels like cortisol. This promotes relaxation and helps alleviate the effects of stress and anxiety.

- **Mind-Body Connection:** Breathing is a powerful link between the mind and body. By consciously altering our breath, we can influence our mental and emotional states. Calm and intentional breathing can help us manage emotions, reduce anxiety, and enhance focus and clarity.

- **Heart Rate Variability (HRV):** HRV is the variation in time intervals between consecutive heartbeats. Higher HRV is associated with better stress resilience and overall health. Slow and deep breathing can increase HRV, indicating a balanced and adaptable autonomic nervous system.

- **Mindfulness and Meditation:** Breathing is a central focus in mindfulness practices and meditation. Paying attention to the breath helps anchor the mind to the present moment and cultivates a state of awareness, reducing mental chatter and promoting a sense of calm.

- **Emotional Regulation:** Breathing techniques can aid in emotional regulation by activating the PNS and calming the nervous system. This can be particularly beneficial during moments of heightened emotions or stress.

Given this profound connection between breath and the nervous system, intentional breathing practices, such as deep breathing exercises, diaphragmatic breathing, and pranayama (controlled breathing techniques from yoga), can be powerful tools to manage stress, promote relaxation, and improve overall well-being. Incorporating these techniques into your daily routine can support a healthier balance between the sympathetic and parasympathetic nervous systems, contributing to a calmer and more resilient mind and body.

## *Breathing Exercises To Induce Relaxation And Alleviate Anxiety Before Bedtime*

Before bedtime, practicing breathing exercises can help induce relaxation, calm the mind, and alleviate anxiety, promoting better sleep. Here are some simple breathing exercises to try:

- **4-7-8 Breathing:**
    a. Sit or lie down comfortably in bed.

    b. Inhale deeply through your nose to a count of 4.

    c. Hold your breath for a count of 7.

    d. Exhale slowly and completely through your mouth to a count of 8.

    e. Repeat this cycle for a few rounds, gradually increasing the duration if comfortable.

    f. This breathing exercise helps slow down your heart rate and encourages relaxation.

- **Diaphragmatic Breathing (Deep Belly Breathing):**
    a. Lie down comfortably on your back in bed or sit with your back straight.

    b. Place one hand on your chest and the other on your abdomen.

    c. Inhale deeply through your nose, allowing your abdomen to rise as you fill your lungs with air. Make sure your chest stays relatively still.

    d. Exhale slowly and completely through your mouth, feeling your abdomen fall as you release the air.

    e. Focus on the sensation of your breath, and continue this deep belly breathing for a few minutes.

    f. This exercise helps calm the nervous system and promotes relaxation.

- **Visualization Breathing:**
  a. Lie down comfortably in bed with your eyes closed.

  b. As you inhale slowly and deeply through your nose, imagine breathing in a calming and soothing light or color.

  c. As you exhale through your mouth, visualize releasing any tension, stress, or anxious thoughts as dark clouds dissipate.

  d. Continue this visualization with each breath, focusing on the peaceful image of inhaling light and exhaling darkness.

  e. This exercise combines deep breathing with calming mental imagery to promote relaxation.

- **Equal Breathing (Sama Vritti):**
  a. Sit comfortably in bed with your spine straight.

  b. Inhale slowly and deeply through your nose to a count of 4.

  c. Exhale through your nose for the same count of 4.

  d. Continue this pattern of equal inhales and exhales, maintaining a steady and relaxed rhythm.

  e. Equal breathing helps create balance and steadiness, calming the mind and body.

- **Humming Bee Breath (Bhramari Pranayama):**
  a. Find a comfortable seated position in bed with your eyes closed.

  b. Place your thumbs on your ears and your index

       fingers over your closed eyes.

c. Inhale deeply through your nose.

d. As you exhale, make a soft humming sound like a bee, allowing the vibrations to resonate in your head.

e. Repeat this process for a few rounds, focusing on the calming effect of the humming sound.

f. Bhramari Pranayama can help release tension and anxiety, promoting relaxation.

Before bedtime, aim to practice these breathing exercises in a calm and quiet environment. You can choose one or a combination of exercises that resonate with you. Consistency is essential; make it a part of your nightly routine to signal your body and mind that it's time to unwind and prepare for sleep. The breathing exercises will help you relax, let go of any anxious thoughts, and create a peaceful transition into a restful night's sleep.

## *Incorporating Breathwork Into Daily Routines To Manage Stress*

Incorporating breathwork into daily routines is a practical and effective way to manage stress and promote overall well-being. By integrating simple breathing exercises throughout your day, you can create moments of calm and relaxation, reduce anxiety, and build resilience to stress. Here are some tips to help you make breathwork a regular part of your daily routine:

**1. Morning Breathing Practice:**

Start your day with a brief breathing exercise to set a positive tone for the day ahead. A few minutes of deep belly breathing or 4-7-8 breathing can help you feel centered and grounded.

**2. Breath Breaks Throughout the Day:**

Take short breath breaks during the day to reset your mind and body. Pause for a few moments to practice deep breathing before or after a stressful meeting, during a work break, or when you feel overwhelmed.

**3. Breathing with Activities:**

Incorporate breathwork into your daily activities. For example, practice diaphragmatic breathing while walking, cooking, or waiting in line. This can help you stay present and reduce tension in your body.

**4. Lunchtime Breathing Session:**

Dedicate a few minutes during your lunch break for a longer breathwork session. Find a quiet space to sit comfortably and practice a breathing exercise of your choice.

**5. Breathing before Bedtime:**

End your day with a calming breathwork practice to wind down and prepare for sleep. Breathing exercises like 4-7-8 or visualization breathing can be especially beneficial before bedtime.

## 6. Breathing during Commute:

Use your commute time to practice breathwork if you're not driving. Breathing exercises can help you relax during busy or stressful commutes.

## 12. Reminder Alarms or Apps:

Set reminders on your phone or use meditation and breathwork apps to prompt you to take breathing breaks throughout the day.

## 13. Breathwork during Work Breaks:

Take advantage of breaks during work or study to practice deep breathing. This can help you refresh your mind and stay focused.

## 14. Breathing before Challenging Tasks:

Take a moment to practice deep breathing before tackling demanding tasks or situations. This can help reduce stress and enhance focus.

## 15. Gratitude Breathing:

Combine gratitude with breathwork by focusing on things you're grateful for while you breathe. This can enhance positive emotions and reduce stress.

Remember that breathwork doesn't require a lot of time; even a few minutes of intentional breathing can have a positive impact on your stress levels. The key is consistency and making breathwork a habit. By incorporating these practices into your daily routine, you can build greater resilience to stress, maintain a calmer state of mind, and improve your overall well-being.

# CHAPTER 5: PREPARING YOUR SLEEP ENVIRONMENT

Preparing your sleep environment is essential for creating a peaceful and conducive space for quality sleep. Your surroundings can significantly impact your ability to fall asleep, stay asleep, and achieve restful slumber. Here are some tips to optimize your sleep environment:

- **Keep It Dark:**
    a. Use blackout curtains or blinds to block out external light sources, especially if you live in a brightly lit area or have street lights outside your window.

    b. Remove or cover any electronic devices with LED displays, as even small amounts of light can disrupt sleep.

- **Keep It Quiet:**
    a. Minimize noise disturbances by using earplugs or a white noise machine to mask disruptive sounds.

    b. Consider soundproofing your room if outside noises are a constant issue.

- **Comfortable Bedding:**
    a. Invest in a comfortable and supportive mattress that suits your preferred sleep position.

    b. Choose pillows and bedding that provide adequate support and temperature regulation for your comfort.

- **Temperature Control:**

      a. Keep your bedroom cool and well-ventilated. The ideal sleep temperature is typically between 60 to 67 degrees Fahrenheit (15 to 19 degrees Celsius).

      b. Use a fan or air conditioner if needed to maintain a comfortable sleeping temperature.

- **Limit Electronic Devices:**

      a. Avoid using electronic devices like smartphones, tablets, and computers in bed, especially before bedtime. The blue light emitted by these devices can disrupt melatonin production and interfere with sleep.

- **Create a Relaxing Atmosphere:**

      a. Decorate your bedroom in soothing colors.

      b. Incorporate relaxing elements like soft lighting, scented candles, or essential oil diffusers with lavender or chamomile scents.

- **Declutter Your Space:**

      a. Keep your sleep environment tidy and free of clutter to create a more peaceful atmosphere.

      b. A clean and organized space can promote a sense of calm and reduce feelings of stress.

- **Limit Bedroom Activities:**

      a. Reserve your bedroom primarily for sleep and intimacy. Avoid working, watching TV, or engaging in stimulating activities in bed.

- **Create a Bedtime Routine:**
     a. Establish a consistent bedtime routine to signal to your body that it's time to wind down and prepare for sleep.

     b. Include relaxing activities such as reading, listening to calming music, or practicing meditation before bed.

By implementing these tips and personalizing your sleep environment to suit your preferences, you can create a space that promotes relaxation and fosters restful sleep. A calming and comfortable sleep environment can significantly improve your sleep quality and overall well-being.

## Creating A Sleep-Conducive Bedroom Atmosphere

Creating a sleep-conducive bedroom atmosphere is essential for promoting relaxation, comfort, and restful sleep. Your bedroom environment plays a significant role in your sleep quality and overall well-being. Here are some tips to create a sleep-friendly atmosphere in your bedroom:

- **Choose Calming Colors:** Opt for soft, neutral, or cool colors on the walls and bedding. Colors like blue, green, or lavender can create a soothing and relaxing ambiance.

- **Comfortable Bedding:** Invest in a comfortable mattress, pillows, and bedding that support your preferred sleep position and keep you at a comfortable temperature throughout the night.

- **Keep It Dark:** Use blackout curtains or shades to block out external light sources, especially if your bedroom receives a lot of natural light or is exposed to streetlights.

- **Limit Noise:** Use earplugs or a white noise machine to mask disruptive sounds and create a peaceful sleep environment. Consider soundproofing your room if necessary.

- **Keep It Cool:** Maintain a cool and comfortable temperature in your bedroom. The ideal sleep temperature is typically between 60 to 67 degrees Fahrenheit (15 to 19 degrees Celsius).

- **Limit Electronic Devices:** Keep electronic devices like smartphones, tablets, and computers out of the bedroom, especially before bedtime. The blue light emitted by these devices can interfere with melatonin production and disrupt sleep.

- **Declutter and Organize:** Keep your bedroom tidy and

free of clutter to create a calming atmosphere. A clean and organized space can promote relaxation and reduce stress.

- **Limit Bedroom Activities:** Reserve your bedroom primarily for sleep and intimacy. Avoid working, watching TV, or engaging in stimulating activities in bed.

- **Create a Relaxing Ambiance:** Incorporate elements that promote relaxation, such as soft lighting, scented candles, or essential oil diffusers with calming scents like lavender or chamomile.

- **Avoid Bright Alarm Clocks:** If you use an alarm clock, choose one with a dim or adjustable display, so it doesn't emit too much light during the night.

- **Implement a Bedtime Routine:** Establish a consistent bedtime routine to signal to your body that it's time to wind down and prepare for sleep. Engage in relaxing activities like reading, gentle stretching, or listening to calming music.

- **Keep Clocks out of Sight:** Place clocks where you cannot easily see them from your bed. Constantly checking the time can create anxiety and disrupt sleep.

- **Promote Fresh Air:** Keep your bedroom well-ventilated to ensure a steady flow of fresh air.

By following these tips, you can transform your bedroom into a peaceful and sleep-conducive space, helping you achieve better sleep quality and overall well-being. Consistency is key, so try to maintain these habits as part of your nightly routine for the best results.

## *Tips For Reducing Noise And Light Disturbances*

Reducing noise and light disturbances in your sleep environment is crucial for promoting better sleep quality and overall restfulness. Here are some tips to help minimize disruptions and create a more serene sleeping space:

**Reducing Noise Disturbances:**

- Use White Noise or Earplugs: Consider using a white noise machine or a fan to create a constant, soothing sound that masks disruptive noises. Alternatively, try using earplugs to block out unwanted sounds.

- Soundproof Your Room: If external noises are a constant issue, consider soundproofing your bedroom. You can use weatherstripping, draft stoppers, or acoustic panels to minimize sound penetration.

- Choose a Quieter Sleep Location: If possible, choose a bedroom that is away from busy streets, noisy neighbors, or other sources of loud sounds.

- Close Windows and Doors: Keep windows and doors closed to reduce outside noise, especially during nighttime hours when the environment is generally quieter.

- Address Household Noises: Identify and address sources of noise within your home, such as noisy appliances or plumbing, and consider making changes to minimize these disturbances.

**Minimizing Light Disturbances:**

- Invest in Blackout Curtains or Blinds: Blackout curtains or blinds can effectively block external light sources, such as streetlights, car headlights, or early morning sunlight.

- Cover Electronic Displays: Cover or dim the displays of electronic devices like clocks, televisions, or smartphones, as even small amounts of light can disrupt sleep.

- Use Sleep Masks: Consider using a comfortable sleep mask to block out light entirely, especially if you're unable to control external light sources.

- Seal Light Leaks: Check for any gaps or cracks around windows and doors that may allow light to seep into your bedroom, and use weatherstripping or blackout materials to seal them.

- Dim Lights Before Bed: In the hour before bedtime, dim the lights in your home to signal your body that it's time to wind down and prepare for sleep.

**Other Tips for a Serene Sleep Environment:**

- Keep Electronics Out of the Bedroom: Limit the use of electronic devices in the bedroom, especially before bedtime. The blue light emitted by screens can interfere with the production of the sleep hormone melatonin.

- Create a Relaxing Bedtime Routine: Establish a consistent bedtime routine that includes calming activities like reading, gentle stretching, or practicing relaxation techniques.

- Maintain a Comfortable Temperature: Keep your bedroom cool and well-ventilated. The ideal sleep temperature is usually between 60 to 67 degrees Fahrenheit (15 to 19 degrees Celsius).

By implementing these tips, you can create a sleep environment that is conducive to restful sleep, helping you wake up feeling refreshed and revitalized each morning. Remember that a peaceful sleep environment is an essential aspect of a healthy sleep routine, and small adjustments can make a big difference in improving your overall sleep quality.

## The Role Of Aromatherapy And Soothing Sounds In Promoting Sleep

Aromatherapy and soothing sounds can play a significant role in promoting sleep and enhancing overall sleep quality. These natural approaches are non-invasive and can create a calming environment, which helps relax the mind and body, making it easier to fall asleep and stay asleep. Here's how aromatherapy and soothing sounds contribute to better sleep:

**Aromatherapy:** Aromatherapy involves using essential oils derived from plants to promote physical and emotional well-being. Essential oils have unique aromatic compounds that can affect the limbic system, the part of the brain associated with emotions and memory. Here's how aromatherapy can promote sleep:

- Calming Effects: Certain essential oils, such as lavender, chamomile, and bergamot, have relaxing properties that can help reduce stress and anxiety, creating a conducive environment for sleep.

- Stress Reduction: Aromatherapy can lower cortisol levels (the stress hormone) and promote the release of calming neurotransmitters like serotonin, helping to ease tension and induce relaxation.

- Enhanced Sleep Quality: Inhaling soothing scents can positively impact sleep quality, making it more restful and reducing nighttime awakenings.

- Sleep Association: Consistently using specific scents during bedtime can create a sleep association, conditioning the brain to associate the aroma with relaxation and sleep.

- Ease of Use: Aromatherapy is easy to incorporate into your bedtime routine. You can use a diffuser, diluted essential oils, or a pillow spray to enjoy the calming scents before sleep.

**Soothing Sounds:** Soothing sounds are gentle and repetitive sounds that help drown out disruptive noises and create a tranquil sleep environment. Here's how soothing sounds can promote better sleep:

- Masking Disruptive Noises: White noise, nature sounds, or ambient music can mask background noises, reducing disturbances that might otherwise wake you up during the night.

- Stress Reduction: Listening to soothing sounds can trigger the relaxation response, lowering stress levels and promoting a sense of calm before sleep.

- Establishing a Sleep Routine: Using consistent soothing sounds during bedtime can serve as a cue for the body to prepare for sleep, helping establish a sleep routine.

- Mind Diversion: Soothing sounds can distract your mind from racing thoughts and worries, allowing you to drift off more easily.

- Improved Sleep Quality: By promoting relaxation and reducing interruptions, soothing sounds can lead to improved sleep quality and a more refreshing sleep experience.

Common soothing sounds include white noise, gentle rainfall, ocean waves, soft instrumental music, and nature sounds like birds chirping or a flowing stream.

Combining aromatherapy and soothing sounds can create a powerful bedtime ritual that prepares both the mind and body for a night of restful sleep. As with any sleep-promoting technique, individual responses may vary, so it's essential to find what works best for you and incorporate these practices consistently into your sleep routine.

# CHAPTER 6: DIGITAL DETOX: MANAGING SCREEN TIME FOR BETTER SLEEP

Managing screen time and implementing a digital detox is crucial for better sleep and overall well-being. The excessive use of electronic devices, such as smartphones, tablets, computers, and televisions, can negatively impact sleep quality and disrupt the body's natural sleep-wake cycle. Here are some tips to help you manage screen time and improve your sleep:

- **Set Screen-Free Hours Before Bed:** Establish a designated period before bedtime where you avoid using electronic devices. Ideally, aim for at least an hour of screen-free time before sleep.

- **Create a Bedtime Routine:** Develop a calming bedtime routine that does not involve screens. Engage in relaxing activities such as reading a book, meditating, or practicing gentle stretching to signal your body that it's time to wind down.

- **Limit Screen Exposure in the Bedroom:** Keep electronic devices out of the bedroom, especially while you are preparing to sleep. This helps create a sleep-conducive environment free from distractions.

- **Use Night Mode or Blue Light Filters:** If you need to

use screens closer to bedtime, enable night mode or blue light filters on your devices. These settings reduce the amount of blue light emitted, which can interfere with melatonin production and disrupt sleep.

- **Set Screen Time Limits:** Use screen time monitoring apps or features built into devices to set daily limits on screen usage. This helps you become more aware of your screen time habits and encourages mindful usage.

- **Avoid Screens in the Middle of the Night:** If you wake up during the night, avoid using screens as they can stimulate your brain and make it harder to fall back asleep. Instead, try relaxation techniques or simply lie quietly in the dark.

- **Designate Tech-Free Zones:** Create specific areas in your home where screens are not allowed, such as the dining table and the bedroom.

- **Use an Analog Alarm Clock:** Replace your smartphone alarm with an analog alarm clock. This eliminates the temptation to use your phone right before bed and upon waking up.

- **Practice the 20-20-20 Rule:** If you spend extended periods looking at screens during the day, follow the 20-20-20 rule. Every 20 minutes, take a 20-second break to look at something 20 feet away. This can help reduce eye strain and fatigue.

- **Explore Screen-Free Hobbies:** Find activities that don't involve screens, such as hobbies, exercise, spending time in nature, or engaging in creative pursuits.

By implementing these strategies and reducing screen time before bedtime, you can improve your sleep quality, fall asleep more easily, and wake up feeling more refreshed. A digital detox can also have positive effects on your overall health and well-being, including reduced stress and increased focus and productivity during the day.

## *Understanding The Impact Of Screens On Sleep Quality*

The impact of screens on sleep quality is significant, and excessive screen time, especially before bedtime, can have negative effects on your sleep. Here are some key ways screens can influence sleep:

- **Blue Light Exposure:** Screens emit blue light, which can suppress the production of the sleep hormone melatonin. Melatonin is essential for regulating the sleep-wake cycle, and its suppression can make it more challenging to fall asleep and disrupt the overall quality of sleep.

- **Delayed Bedtime:** Engaging in screen activities, such as watching TV shows, playing video games, or using social media, can be stimulating and lead to delayed bedtime. This cuts into your sleep time and may result in sleep deprivation.

- **Sleep Fragmentation:** Using screens close to bedtime can lead to sleep fragmentation, meaning your sleep becomes more fragmented with more awakenings during the night. This can reduce the overall duration of deep, restorative sleep.

- **Heightened Arousal and Stress:** Exposure to stimulating content, such as intense movies or stressful news, can lead to increased arousal and stress before bed. This heightened state of alertness can interfere with your ability to relax and fall asleep.

- **Sleep Onset Insomnia:** The blue light from screens can delay the onset of sleep, leading to a condition called sleep onset insomnia. It may take longer for you to fall asleep, and this can negatively impact the overall duration and quality of your sleep.

- **Cognitive Stimulation:** Engaging in mentally

stimulating activities on screens can keep your mind active and alert, making it harder to transition into a state of relaxation required for sleep.

- **Decreased Sleep Duration:** The use of screens late at night can lead to a delay in bedtime and result in a decrease in overall sleep duration, leading to sleep deprivation over time.

- **Impact on Circadian Rhythm:** Exposure to screens in the evening can disrupt the body's natural circadian rhythm, which regulates sleep and wake cycles. This disruption can lead to irregular sleep patterns and difficulties maintaining a consistent sleep schedule.

To improve sleep quality, it's essential to limit screen time, especially in the hour or two before bedtime. Creating a screen-free wind-down routine and engaging in relaxing activities can help signal your body that it's time to sleep. If you need to use screens closer to bedtime, consider using blue light filters or night mode to minimize the impact of blue light on melatonin production. Ultimately, reducing screen time and adopting healthy sleep habits can lead to more restful and rejuvenating sleep.

## *Strategies To Limit Screen Time Before Bedtime*

Limiting screen time before bedtime is crucial for improving sleep quality and promoting a restful night. Here are some effective strategies to help you reduce screen time and create a more sleep-friendly routine:

- **Set a Screen Curfew:** Establish a specific time in the evening when you will stop using screens. Aim to have a screen curfew at least one hour before your intended bedtime.

- **Create a Bedtime Routine:** Develop a calming bedtime routine that does not involve screens. Engage in relaxing activities such as reading a book, practicing gentle yoga or stretching, or listening to soothing music.

- **Charge Devices Outside the Bedroom:** Keep electronic devices like smartphones and tablets out of the bedroom during sleep hours. Charge them in another room or at a distance where you won't be tempted to check them right before bed.

- **Use an Alarm Clock:** Replace your smartphone's alarm with a traditional alarm clock. This prevents the need to use your phone just before sleep and upon waking up.

- **Prepare for the Next Day Earlier:** Finish any necessary work or tasks involving screens well before bedtime, so you're not tempted to use screens right up until sleep time.

- **Avoid Stimulating Content:** Refrain from watching intense, action-packed, or emotionally stimulating content before bedtime. Instead, choose calming and uplifting activities.

- **Dim the Lights:** Lower the brightness of screens during the evening and consider using blue light filters or night mode settings to reduce the impact of blue light on melatonin production.

- **Set App Limits and Notifications:** Use app settings on your phone to set daily time limits for specific apps. You can also disable non-essential notifications in the evening to reduce screen distractions.

- **Prioritize Wind-Down Time:** Allocate time in the evening for relaxation and reflection. Engage in activities that promote calmness and peace of mind.

- **Practice Mindfulness or Meditation:** Consider practicing mindfulness or meditation before bedtime to help clear your mind and prepare for sleep.

- **Use Technology Wisely:** If you must use screens in the evening, choose activities that are relaxing and less stimulating, such as listening to soothing music or engaging in a guided meditation.

- **Involve Your Household:** Encourage other household members to limit screen time before bedtime. A supportive environment can make it easier for everyone to adopt healthier sleep habits.

By implementing these strategies, you can gradually reduce your screen time before bedtime and create a more conducive sleep environment. Consistency is key, so stick to your new routine to allow your body to adjust and improve your overall sleep quality. Remember that quality sleep is essential for physical and mental well-being, and limiting screen time is a simple yet effective way to support better sleep.

## *Alternative Activities To Relax And Unwind In The Evening*

There are plenty of alternative activities to help you relax and unwind in the evening without relying on screens. Here are some calming and enjoyable options:

- **Reading:** Pick up a good book or magazine and immerse yourself in a captivating story or informative content.

- **Journaling:** Write down your thoughts, feelings, or reflections in a journal. Journaling can be a therapeutic way to process your day and clear your mind before bedtime.

- **Listening to Music:** Create a playlist of soothing and calming music to listen to in the evening. Instrumental music, classical tunes, or nature sounds can be particularly relaxing.

- **Practicing Yoga or Stretching:** Engage in gentle yoga or stretching exercises to release tension and promote relaxation.

- **Meditation:** Practice mindfulness or meditation to quiet your mind and reduce stress. Meditation can help you find inner peace and prepare for sleep.

- **Aromatherapy:** Use essential oils or scented candles with calming fragrances like lavender or chamomile to create a serene atmosphere.

- **Taking a Bath:** Enjoy a warm bath with Epsom salts or bath oils to relax your muscles and calm your mind.

- **Drinking Herbal Tea:** Sip on caffeine-free herbal teas like chamomile, valerian root, or passionflower, which are known for their calming properties.

- **Engaging in Hobbies:** Pursue hobbies that bring you joy and relaxation, such as drawing, painting, knitting, or crafting.

- **Nature Walk or Stargazing:** Spend some time outdoors, taking a leisurely walk in nature or stargazing to connect with the peacefulness of the night sky.

- **Deep Breathing Exercises:** Practice deep breathing or relaxation techniques to ease stress and promote tranquility.

- **Gentle Exercise:** Consider gentle exercises like tai chi or qigong, which can help you find balance and relaxation.

- **Spending Quality Time with Loved Ones:** Engage in meaningful conversations or spend quality time with family members or friends.

- **Savoring a Warm Drink:** Enjoy a warm and calming drink like warm milk or herbal tea as you wind down.

- **Creating Art:** Engage in artistic activities like drawing, coloring, or crafting, which can be meditative and soothing.

Remember, the goal of these activities is to help you unwind and create a peaceful environment before bedtime. Choose activities that resonate with you and make them a part of your evening routine to signal your body and mind that it's time to relax and prepare for a restful night's sleep.

# CHAPTER 7: MINDFULNESS TECHNIQUES FOR LETTING GO OF DAILY WORRIES

Mindfulness techniques can be incredibly helpful for letting go of daily worries and promoting a sense of calm and inner peace. Here are some mindfulness practices you can incorporate into your daily routine to release worries and anxieties:

- **Mindful Breathing:** Take a few minutes to focus on your breath. Pay attention to each inhale and exhale, allowing your breath to become slower and deeper. When worries arise, gently bring your focus back to your breath.

- **Body Scan Meditation:** Close your eyes and systematically scan your body from head to toe, noticing any areas of tension or discomfort. Breathe into these areas and consciously release any physical tension, which can help release mental worries as well.

- **Thought Observation:** Observe your thoughts without judgment. When worries arise, acknowledge them, and then let them pass without getting caught up in them. Imagine your thoughts as clouds drift by in the sky.

- **Grounding Techniques:** Connect with the present

moment by using grounding techniques. Feel the sensation of your feet on the ground or notice the texture of an object in your hand. This helps anchor you to the here and now, letting go of worries about the past or future.

- **Mindful Walking:** Take a mindful walk, paying attention to the sensations in your body and the environment around you. Whenever worries surface, gently bring your focus back to the present moment.

- **Gratitude Practice:** Shift your focus from worries to gratitude. Take a moment to acknowledge and appreciate the positive aspects of your life. Cultivating a sense of gratitude can help shift your perspective and reduce worries.

- **Mindful Eating:** Practice mindful eating by savoring each bite of your meal, noticing the flavors, textures, and smells. Engaging your senses in this way can help you stay present and let go of worries.

- **Visualization:** Imagine your worries as leaves floating down a river or clouds drifting away in the sky. Visualize yourself letting go of each worry as you watch them drift away from your awareness.

- **Labeling Your Thoughts:** When worries arise, mentally label them as "thinking" and let them go. Remind yourself that thoughts are temporary and do not define you.

- **Meditation:** Set aside time for meditation regularly. Meditation allows you to observe your thoughts and feelings without attachment, helping you gain a greater sense of inner peace and detachment from worries.

Remember that mindfulness is a practice, and it's okay if your mind wanders or worries still arise. Be gentle with yourself and keep coming back to the present moment. With consistent practice, you'll find it easier to let go of daily worries and cultivate a greater sense of inner calm and acceptance.

## How To Detach From Work And Responsibilities Mentally

Detaching from work and responsibilities mentally is essential for maintaining a healthy work-life balance and preventing burnout. Here are some strategies to help you detach and create boundaries between your work and personal life:

- **Establish Clear Work Hours:** Set specific work hours and stick to them as much as possible. Define a clear start and end time for your workday, and avoid working outside these designated hours.

- **Create a Workspace:** Designate a specific area in your home for work-related activities. When you're done with work, physically leave that space to mentally signal the end of the workday.

- **Turn Off Work Notifications:** Disable work-related notifications on your phone and other devices during non-work hours. This prevents constant interruptions and allows you to fully disconnect from work.

- **Prioritize Breaks:** Schedule regular breaks throughout your workday to rest and recharge. Use these breaks to step away from your work and engage in activities that help you relax.

- **Practice Mindfulness Techniques:** Use mindfulness techniques, such as deep breathing or meditation, to stay present in the moment and avoid getting caught up in work-related thoughts during your time.

- **Create a Transition Ritual:** Develop a ritual that helps you transition from work to personal time. It could be something as simple as closing your laptop, stretching, or going for a short walk.

- **Engage in Hobbies:** Dedicate time to hobbies and

activities that you enjoy and that have nothing to do with work. Engaging in these activities can help take your mind off work-related concerns.

- **Limit Work-Related Conversations:** Try to avoid discussing work matters during your time. Set boundaries with colleagues and let them know when you are available for work-related discussions.

- **Set Realistic Expectations:** Understand that it's okay to take time for yourself and that you don't need to be constantly available for work. Set realistic expectations for yourself and others regarding your availability outside of work hours.

- **Practice Self-Compassion:** Be kind to yourself and recognize that it's natural to have work-related thoughts and worries. Instead of being critical, practice self-compassion and remind yourself that it's essential to take breaks and disconnect.

- **Plan Personal Activities:** Schedule activities or outings during your time that you look forward to. Having enjoyable plans can motivate you to detach from work and fully engage in your personal life.

- **Delegate and Seek Support:** Learn to delegate tasks when possible and seek support from colleagues or superiors when you need it. Knowing that you have support can help ease the pressure and reduce work-related mental clutter.

By implementing these strategies, you can create a healthier boundary between work and personal life, allowing you to be fully detached mentally from work and enjoy your time more fully. Remember that work is just one aspect of your life, and taking care of your well-being requires maintaining a balance that includes time for relaxation, personal interests, and meaningful connections with loved ones.

## *Practicing Mindfulness To Avoid Rumination Before Bedtime*

Practicing mindfulness before bedtime can be a powerful tool to avoid rumination and promote a peaceful and restful night's sleep. Rumination, the act of repetitively focusing on negative thoughts and feelings, can keep your mind active and hinder your ability to relax and fall asleep. Here's how mindfulness can help you let go of rumination and prepare for better sleep:

- **Mindful Breathing:** Engage in deep breathing exercises to shift your focus away from rumination. Pay attention to the sensations of your breath as you inhale and exhale, allowing it to become slower and more rhythmic.

- **Body Scan Meditation:** Perform a body scan, slowly bringing your attention to different parts of your body, starting from your toes and moving upward. This helps you become aware of any tension and release physical and mental stress.

- **Thought Observation:** Practice observing your thoughts without judgment. When ruminative thoughts arise, acknowledge them, but avoid getting entangled in the content. Let the thoughts pass like clouds drifting by in the sky.

- **Grounding Techniques:** Ground yourself in the present moment by focusing on your senses. Notice the feeling of your body on the bed, the sounds around you, or the feeling of your breath. This anchors you to the present, preventing rumination about the past or worries about the future.

- **Acceptance and Letting Go:** Instead of trying to suppress or control your thoughts, practice acceptance. Acknowledge that ruminative thoughts may arise, but remind yourself that they don't define you, and they will pass with time.

- **Visualization:** Visualize a peaceful and serene place in your mind, such as a calming beach or a beautiful forest. Immerse yourself in the details of this place to distract your mind from rumination.

- **Gratitude Practice:** Shift your focus from negative thoughts to gratitude. Take a moment to reflect on things you are grateful for, helping shift your perspective to a more positive mindset.

- **Journaling:** If persistent thoughts are keeping you awake, consider writing them down in a journal before bedtime. This act of externalizing your thoughts can help release them from your mind.

- **Mindful Movement:** Engage in gentle and mindful movement exercises like stretching or yoga. These activities help release tension and promote relaxation, diverting your mind from rumination.

- **Limit Pre-Sleep Stimuli:** Avoid engaging in stimulating activities or having intense discussions before bedtime. Instead, choose calming and soothing activities to prepare your mind for sleep.

By incorporating mindfulness practices into your evening routine, you can let go of rumination, reduce anxiety, and cultivate a more peaceful and relaxed state of mind. Consistency is key; the more you practice mindfulness, the more effective it becomes in helping you break the cycle of rumination and promote better sleep.

## *Cultivating A Positive Mindset For Better Sleep Outcomes*

Cultivating a positive mindset can significantly impact your sleep outcomes and overall well-being. A positive mindset can help reduce stress, anxiety, and negative thoughts that often disrupt sleep. Here are some strategies to foster a positive mindset for better sleep:

- **Practice Gratitude:** Regularly take time to reflect on the things you are grateful for in your life. Keeping a gratitude journal or simply listing a few things you are thankful for each day can shift your focus from negativity to positivity.

- **Positive Affirmations:** Use positive affirmations to challenge and replace negative thoughts. Repeat positive statements to yourself, such as "I am calm and at peace," "I am capable of handling any challenges," or "I am deserving of a good night's sleep."

- **Focus on Solutions:** When faced with challenges or problems, try to shift your focus from dwelling on the negatives to seeking solutions. A problem-solving mindset can reduce feelings of helplessness and improve overall well-being.

- **Surround Yourself with Positivity:** Spend time with positive and supportive people who uplift and inspire you. Engage in activities that bring you joy and happiness.

- **Limit Negative Media Exposure:** Be mindful of the media content you consume, especially before bedtime. Avoid exposure to negative news or disturbing content that may cause stress or anxiety.

- **Visualize Positive Outcomes:** Use visualization techniques to imagine positive and relaxing scenarios before bedtime. Create mental images of a peaceful environment, a restful night's sleep, or successful outcomes in your daily life.

- **Practice Mindfulness and Meditation:** Engage in mindfulness practices and meditation to become more aware of your thoughts and emotions. This helps you let go of negative thought patterns and fosters a more positive outlook.

- **Celebrate Small Wins:** Acknowledge and celebrate your accomplishments, no matter how small they may seem. Recognizing your achievements can boost your confidence and overall mood.

- **Engage in Positive Self-Talk:** Replace self-criticism with self-compassion and positive self-talk. Treat yourself with the same kindness and understanding you would offer to a friend.

- **Set Realistic Goals:** Set achievable and realistic goals for yourself. Celebrate progress and acknowledge that setbacks are a normal part of life's journey.

- **Limit Social Comparison:** Avoid comparing yourself to others, especially on social media. Focus on your own growth and progress without constantly measuring yourself against others.

- **Practice Random Acts of Kindness:** Engage in acts of kindness towards others, as this can bring a sense of fulfillment and positivity to your life.

By cultivating a positive mindset, you can create a more favorable mental environment that supports better sleep outcomes. Incorporate these strategies into your daily life, especially before bedtime, to shift your focus from negativity to positivity and enjoy the benefits of improved sleep and overall well-being.

# CHAPTER 8: BEDTIME YOGA FOR RELAXATION

Bedtime yoga can be a wonderful way to unwind and relax before going to sleep. These gentle and calming yoga poses can help release tension from the body and quiet the mind, promoting better sleep and a more restful night. Here is a simple bedtime yoga routine for relaxation:

- **Child's Pose (Balasana):** Start on your hands and knees, then gently sit back on your heels, reaching your arms forward and lowering your chest toward the floor. Hold the pose, breathing deeply and allowing your forehead to rest on the mat. This pose helps to stretch the back and hips, relieving tension.

- **Standing Forward Bend (Uttanasana):** Stand with your feet hip-width apart and slowly fold forward from the hips, letting your upper body hang over your legs. Allow your arms to dangle or hold onto your elbows. This pose releases tension in the hamstrings and lower back.

- **Butterfly Pose (Baddha Konasana):** Sit on the bed and bring the soles of your feet together, letting your knees fall out to the sides. Hold your feet with your hands and gently flap your knees up and down like butterfly wings. This pose opens up the hips and groin area.

- **Supine Twist:** Lie on your back, bring your knees

towards your chest, and then drop them to one side while keeping your shoulders flat on the bed. Extend your arms out to the sides and turn your head in the opposite direction of your knees. Hold for a few breaths and then switch sides. This pose releases tension in the spine and helps to massage the abdominal organs.

- **Legs up the Wall (Viparita Karani):** Sit sideways on your bed and swing your legs up the wall while lying on your back. Your hips should be close to the wall or headboard. This pose is incredibly relaxing and helps to improve circulation.

- **Corpse Pose (Savasana):** Lie flat on your back with your legs slightly apart and your arms relaxed by your sides. Close your eyes and focus on your breath, allowing your body to completely let go of any tension. Stay in this pose for several minutes, clearing your mind and preparing for a peaceful night's sleep.

Remember to breathe deeply and stay in each pose for as long as feels comfortable. Avoid any strenuous or intense poses before bedtime, as they may stimulate the body instead of relaxing it. Take your time and allow yourself to fully relax and unwind with these gentle bedtime yoga poses. Sweet dreams!

## *Gentle Yoga Poses To Release Tension And Prepare The Body For Sleep*

Gentle yoga poses can be incredibly beneficial for releasing tension and preparing the body for sleep. These poses help relax the body and mind, relieve stress, and promote a sense of calmness, making it easier to transition into restful sleep. Here are some gentle yoga poses that you can practice before bedtime:

### 1. Child's Pose (Balasana):

- Kneel on the floor with your big toes touching and knees slightly wider than hip-width apart.

- Sit back on your heels and fold your upper body forward, reaching your arms out in front of you.

- Rest your forehead on the mat and breathe deeply, allowing your spine to lengthen and your hips to relax.

### 2. Standing Forward Bend (Uttanasana):

- Stand with feet hip-width apart and fold your upper body forward, hinging at the hips.

- Let your upper body hang loosely, and allow your head and neck to relax.

- You can bend your knees slightly if you feel any tension in your hamstrings.

### 3. Seated Forward Bend (Paschimottanasana):

- Sit on the floor with your legs extended in front of you.

- Inhale and lengthen your spine, then exhale and fold forward from your hips, reaching for your toes or shins.

- Focus on keeping your back straight and your neck relaxed

as you breathe deeply into the stretch.

### 4. Legs Up the Wall (Viparita Karani):

- Lie on your back with your buttocks close to a wall.

- Extend your legs up the wall, keeping them straight and relaxed.

- You can use a pillow or cushion under your hips for added support and comfort.

### 5. Reclining Bound Angle Pose (Supta Baddha Konasana):

- Lie on your back and bring the soles of your feet together, allowing your knees to open outward.

- Place pillows or cushions under your knees and arms to support your body and help you relax.

### 6. Corpse Pose (Savasana):

- Lie flat on your back with your arms by your sides and palms facing up.

- Close your eyes and focus on deep, slow breaths, allowing your body to fully relax.

- Stay in this pose for several minutes, letting go of any tension or stress.

These gentle yoga poses can be practiced as a bedtime routine to help release physical tension and calm the mind, creating a peaceful transition to sleep. Remember to focus on your breath and avoid any discomfort in the poses. If you have any specific health concerns or conditions, it's a good idea to consult with a yoga instructor or healthcare professional before starting a new yoga practice.

## The Relationship Between Yoga And Sleep Quality

The relationship between yoga and sleep quality is well-established, as yoga can have a positive impact on various aspects of sleep. Regular yoga practice has been shown to improve sleep quality, reduce sleep disturbances, and promote overall sleep health. Here are some ways yoga contributes to better sleep:

- **Stress Reduction:** Yoga incorporates relaxation techniques, deep breathing, and mindfulness practices that help reduce stress and anxiety. By calming the nervous system and promoting relaxation, yoga prepares the body and mind for restful sleep.

- **Mind-Body Connection:** Yoga fosters a better mind-body connection, which can help individuals become more aware of their physical sensations and emotions. This increased awareness can lead to better stress management and improved sleep.

- **Muscle Relaxation:** Many yoga poses involve gentle stretches and muscle relaxation techniques, helping to release tension and ease physical discomfort that might otherwise interfere with sleep.

- **Regulation of the Nervous System:** Certain yoga practices, like restorative or gentle yoga, stimulate the parasympathetic nervous system, which is responsible for the body's "rest and digest" response. This activation helps counteract the effects of the sympathetic nervous system (fight-or-flight response) and promotes relaxation.

- **Breath Control:** Yoga incorporates breath control (pranayama), which can have a calming effect on the mind and body. Deep breathing practices can reduce anxiety and help individuals transition into a more relaxed state before bedtime.

- **Mindfulness and Meditation:** Mindfulness practices and meditation taught in yoga can improve sleep by reducing racing thoughts, promoting present-moment awareness, and decreasing mental agitation.

- **Improved Sleep Efficiency:** Regular yoga practice has been associated with improved sleep efficiency, which means spending a higher percentage of time in bed asleep rather than awake.

- **Reduction of Insomnia Symptoms:** Studies have shown that yoga can be beneficial in reducing symptoms of insomnia, helping individuals fall asleep faster, stay asleep longer, and experience more restorative sleep.

- **Management of Sleep Disorders:** For individuals with certain sleep disorders, such as sleep apnea or restless legs syndrome, yoga may provide complementary support in managing symptoms and improving sleep.

- **Daytime Energy and Alertness:** Better sleep quality from yoga practice can lead to improved daytime energy levels and enhanced overall well-being.

It's important to note that individual responses to yoga and its impact on sleep quality may vary. While yoga can be beneficial for many people, it's essential to find the right type and intensity of practice that suits your needs and preferences. If you have specific sleep concerns or medical conditions, consult with a healthcare professional or a qualified yoga instructor to tailor a practice that supports your sleep health. Incorporating yoga into your routine, especially in the evening, can be a valuable tool for promoting better sleep and overall well-being.

## *Creating A Personalized Bedtime Yoga Routine*

Creating a personalized bedtime yoga routine is a wonderful way to wind down and prepare your body and mind for a restful night's sleep. Here's a step-by-step guide to help you design a bedtime yoga routine tailored to your needs:

- **Set a Relaxing Environment:** Find a quiet and comfortable space in your home where you can practice without distractions. Dim the lights or use soft lighting to create a calming atmosphere.
- **Start with Breath Awareness:** Begin your routine with a few minutes of breath awareness or pranayama. Sit comfortably and focus on slow, deep breaths, inhaling and exhaling through your nose.
- **Gentle Warm-Up Poses:** Start with some gentle warm-up poses to loosen up your body. You can do gentle neck rolls, shoulder rolls, seated twists, and side stretches.
- **Choose Soothing Poses:** Include relaxing poses that encourage tension release. Some examples include:
    a. Child's Pose (Balasana)
    b. Standing Forward Fold (Uttanasana)
    c. Reclining Bound Angle Pose (Supta Baddha Konasana)
    d. Supine Twist (Supta Matsyendrasana)
- **Hold Poses Longer:** Spend more time in each pose than you might during a typical yoga practice. Holding poses for 1-2 minutes allows you to sink deeper into the stretch and experience greater relaxation.
- **Incorporate Restorative Poses:** Consider adding restorative yoga poses that are especially conducive to relaxation. Some restorative poses include:
    a. Legs Up the Wall (Viparita Karani)
    b. Supported Bridge Pose
    c. Supported Child's Pose

d. Supported Reclining Twist

- **End with Savasana:** Conclude your routine with a longer Savasana (Corpse Pose). Lie down on your back, close your eyes, and allow your body to fully relax. Focus on your breath and let go of any remaining tension.
- **Add Meditation or Visualization:** After Savasana, you can include a short meditation or visualization practice. Imagine yourself in a peaceful and calming environment, such as a serene beach or a quiet forest.
- **Create a Routine Length That Works for You:** Depending on your schedule and preferences, aim for a bedtime yoga routine that lasts anywhere from 15 to 30 minutes.
- **Be Consistent:** Commit to practicing your personalized bedtime yoga routine regularly, ideally at the same time each night. Consistency will reinforce the relaxation response and signal to your body that it's time to wind down for sleep.

Remember that your bedtime yoga routine should be gentle and calming, avoiding vigorous or stimulating poses that could disrupt your sleep. Listen to your body and adjust the routine as needed based on how you feel each night. Personalizing your bedtime yoga routine to suit your needs will help you cultivate better sleep habits and promote a deeper sense of relaxation and well-being.

# CHAPTER 9: PROGRESSIVE MUSCLE RELAXATION

Progressive Muscle Relaxation (PMR) is a relaxation technique that involves systematically tensing and relaxing different muscle groups in the body to promote physical and mental relaxation. It's a simple yet effective method for reducing muscle tension, stress, and anxiety, making it an excellent practice for promoting better sleep. Here's how to do Progressive Muscle Relaxation:

**Step-by-Step Guide:**

- **Find a Comfortable Position:** Lie down on your back or sit in a comfortable chair with your feet flat on the ground and your hands resting on your lap.

- **Take Deep Breaths:** Close your eyes and take a few deep breaths to center yourself and become aware of your body.

- **Start with the Toes:** Focus on your toes and deliberately tense the muscles in that area. Curl your toes tightly and hold the tension for about 5-10 seconds.

- **Release the Tension:** Suddenly let go of the tension and relax the muscles completely, feeling the sensations of relaxation in your toes. Pay attention to the contrast between tension and relaxation.

- **Move Up the Body:** Continue the process by moving

up the body. Tense and release each muscle group sequentially, holding the tension for 5-10 seconds before relaxing.

    a. Feet and calves

    b. Thighs and buttocks

    c. Abdomen

    d. Hands and forearms

    e. Upper arms and shoulders

    f. Neck and jaw

    g. Face (squint your eyes and tense your facial muscles)

- **Focus on Breath:** Throughout the practice, maintain slow, deep breathing. Inhale as you tense the muscles, and exhale as you release the tension.

- **Scan for Tension:** If you notice any residual tension in a specific area, repeat the tensing and relaxing process for that muscle group.

- **End with Full Relaxation:** After completing the muscle groups, take a few moments to relax your entire body. Imagine a wave of relaxation washing over you, releasing any remaining tension.

- **Stay in the Relaxed State:** Spend a few minutes in this deeply relaxed state, enjoying the feeling of tranquility and calmness.

Progressive Muscle Relaxation can be practiced at any time during the day, but it's particularly beneficial before bedtime to prepare your body and mind for sleep. Consistent practice can help reduce muscle tension, alleviate stress, and promote better sleep quality. As with any relaxation technique, the more you practice, the more effective it becomes, so consider incorporating PMR into your nightly routine for the best results.

## Introduction To Progressive Muscle Relaxation As A Technique For Deep Relaxation

Progressive Muscle Relaxation (PMR) is a widely used relaxation technique designed to induce a state of deep relaxation in both the body and mind. It was developed by American physician and psychologist Edmund Jacobson in the early 20th century. PMR involves systematically tensing and relaxing different muscle groups to help individuals become more aware of muscle tension and learn to release it intentionally.

The primary goal of PMR is to reduce physical and mental tension, stress, and anxiety. By practicing PMR regularly, individuals can experience a profound sense of relaxation, which can have numerous benefits for overall well-being, including improved sleep quality, reduced muscle pain, and enhanced emotional well-being.

**How Progressive Muscle Relaxation Works:**

During PMR, you learn to tense specific muscle groups for a brief period (typically 5-10 seconds) and then release the tension, allowing the muscles to relax completely. By deliberately tensing and releasing the muscles, you can become more aware of the physical sensations associated with tension and relaxation.

The sequence of tensing and relaxing muscle groups helps to:

- **Increase Body Awareness:** PMR helps you become more in tune with the different areas of your body and the sensations they generate.

- **Reduce Muscle Tension:** The intentional release of muscle tension helps to alleviate physical tightness and discomfort.

- **Activate the Relaxation Response:** The relaxation response is the body's natural counterpart to the stress response. PMR activates the parasympathetic nervous system, which calms the body and promotes relaxation.

- **Quiet the Mind:** Focusing on muscle tension and relaxation distracts the mind from worrisome thoughts, allowing for a mental break.

**Benefits of Progressive Muscle Relaxation:**

- Stress Reduction: PMR is an effective tool for managing stress and anxiety, helping to promote a sense of calm and inner peace.

- By reducing physical tension and mental stress, PMR can improve sleep patterns and enhance sleep quality.

- Muscle Pain Relief: Improved Sleep Quality: Regular practice of PMR can alleviate muscle pain and discomfort associated with tension and stress.

- Emotional Well-Being: PMR can help individuals manage emotional challenges, such as anger, frustration, and irritability, by promoting a more relaxed state of mind.

- Enhanced Focus and Concentration: A relaxed mind is better able to focus and concentrate on tasks.

- Lower Blood Pressure: The relaxation response triggered by PMR can lead to a reduction in blood pressure levels.

**Getting Started with Progressive Muscle Relaxation:**

You can practice PMR on your own using guided instructions or audio recordings, or you can attend a class or session led by a trained instructor. Consistency is essential for experiencing the full benefits of PMR, so incorporating it into your daily or nightly routine is recommended.

Remember that PMR is safe for most people, but if you have any pre-existing medical conditions or concerns, consult with a healthcare professional before starting this or any other relaxation technique. With regular practice, you can cultivate deep relaxation, reduce stress, and enjoy the positive effects of Progressive Muscle Relaxation on your overall well-being.

## *Step-By-Step Guide To Practicing PMR For Better Sleep*

Practicing Progressive Muscle Relaxation (PMR) before bedtime can help you release tension and anxiety, promoting a more relaxed state conducive to better sleep. Here's a step-by-step guide to help you practice PMR for better sleep:

### Step 1: Find a Quiet Space

- Choose a quiet and comfortable place where you won't be disturbed during your PMR practice.

### Step 2: Get Comfortable

- Lie down on your back on a yoga mat or your bed with your arms by your sides and your legs slightly apart. Close your eyes to enhance relaxation.

### Step 3: Take a Few Deep Breaths

- Take a few slow and deep breaths to help you relax and bring your awareness to the present moment.

### Step 4: Begin the Tension-Relaxation Process

- Start with your feet. Curl your toes and tense the muscles in your feet, holding the tension for 5-10 seconds.

### Step 5: Release the Tension

- Suddenly let go of the tension in your feet, allowing them to relax completely. Feel the sensations of relaxation in your feet.

### Step 6: Move Up the Body

- Progressively move up your body, repeating the tension and relaxation process for each muscle group. Typically, you might tense and relax the following muscle groups:

a. Calves and shins

b. Thighs

c. Hips and buttocks

d. Abdomen

e. Hands and forearms

f. Upper arms and shoulders

g. Neck and jaw

h. Face (squint your eyes and tense your facial muscles)

**Step 7: Focus on Your Breath**

- Throughout the practice, maintain slow, deep breathing. Inhale as you tense the muscles and exhale as you release the tension.

**Step 8: Pay Attention to Sensations**

- As you tense and relax each muscle group, pay attention to the sensations in your body. Notice the difference between tension and relaxation.

**Step 9: Repeat or Stay in the Final Relaxation**

- After completing the tension-relaxation process for all muscle groups, you can choose to repeat the entire sequence or spend a few minutes in the final relaxation.

**Step 10: Final Relaxation (Savasana)**

- Lie down on your back, allowing your entire body to relax deeply.

- Let go of any remaining tension and simply rest in stillness for a few minutes.

**Step 11: End with Mindfulness**

- When you're ready to conclude your practice, gently

bring your awareness back to your surroundings. Wiggle your fingers and toes, slowly open your eyes, and take a few moments to transition back to your waking state.

## Step 12: Drift into Sleep

- As you lie in bed after your PMR practice, focus on your breath and let go of any thoughts. Allow yourself to drift into sleep naturally.

Consistency is key to experiencing the full benefits of PMR. Aim to practice this relaxation technique regularly, ideally before bedtime, to prepare your body and mind for a peaceful and restful night's sleep. With practice, you'll likely find it easier to release tension and enter a state of deep relaxation, helping you achieve better sleep outcomes.

## Combining PMR With Breathing Exercises And Meditation For Enhanced Results

Combining Progressive Muscle Relaxation (PMR) with breathing exercises and meditation can enhance the overall relaxation experience and promote even deeper levels of calmness, reducing stress and anxiety more effectively. Integrating these practices creates a comprehensive relaxation routine that prepares both the body and mind for better sleep. Here's how to combine PMR, breathing exercises, and meditation for enhanced results:

**Step 1: Find a Quiet Space**

- Choose a quiet and comfortable space where you won't be disturbed during your relaxation practice.

**Step 2: Get Comfortable**

- Lie down on your back on a yoga mat or your bed with your arms by your sides and your legs slightly apart. Close your eyes to enhance relaxation.

**Step 3: Take a Few Deep Breaths**

- Begin with a few rounds of deep breathing to center yourself and bring your awareness to the present moment.

**Step 4: Progressive Muscle Relaxation (PMR)**

- Start with your feet and progressively move up your body, tensing and relaxing each muscle group as described in the PMR practice earlier.

**Step 5: Diaphragmatic Breathing (Deep Belly Breathing)**

- After completing PMR, shift your focus to your breath. Practice diaphragmatic breathing by inhaling deeply through your nose, allowing your belly to rise as you fill your lungs with air.

- Exhale slowly and completely through your nose, feeling your belly fall as you release your breath.

- Continue this deep belly breathing for a few minutes, syncing your breath with a natural and calming rhythm.

## Step 6: Body Scan Meditation

- After the breathing exercises, transition into a body scan meditation. Bring your attention to each part of your body, starting from your toes and moving upward to the crown of your head.

- As you scan each body part, observe any lingering tension or sensations without judgment. Allow yourself to release and let go of any tension you may find.

## Step 7: Mindfulness Meditation

- After the body scan, shift your focus to a mindfulness meditation practice. Observe your thoughts and emotions as they arise without getting attached to them. Imagine them as passing clouds in the sky, allowing them to come and go without interference.

- Whenever your mind wanders, gently guide your attention back to your breath or a specific point of focus.

## Step 8: Final Relaxation (Savasana)

- Conclude your relaxation practice by returning to a state of stillness and rest. Allow yourself to fully relax and let go.

## Step 9: Transition to Sleep

- When you're ready, gently bring your awareness back to your surroundings. Wiggle your fingers and toes, slowly open your eyes, and take a few moments to transition back to your waking state.

By combining PMR with breathing exercises and meditation,

you create a holistic relaxation routine that addresses both the physical and mental aspects of relaxation. This integrated practice can significantly reduce stress and promote a sense of calm, making it an ideal bedtime routine to prepare for a restful night's sleep. Regular practice of this combined relaxation routine can have cumulative benefits, leading to improved sleep quality and overall well-being.

# CHAPTER 10: OVERCOMING SLEEP DISORDERS

Overcoming sleep disorders can be a challenging process, but with the right strategies and support, it is possible to improve sleep quality and regain restful nights. Here are some steps and tips to help you address common sleep disorders:

**1. Identify the Sleep Disorder:** The first step is to recognize and identify the specific sleep disorder you are experiencing. Common sleep disorders include insomnia, sleep apnea, restless legs syndrome (RLS), narcolepsy, and sleepwalking, among others. Consulting a healthcare professional or a sleep specialist is essential for a proper diagnosis.

**2. Seek Professional Help:** If you suspect you have a sleep disorder, consult a healthcare professional or a sleep specialist. They can conduct a thorough evaluation, which may involve a sleep study (polysomnography) or other assessments, to diagnose the condition accurately.

**3. Follow Treatment Recommendations:** Once diagnosed, follow the treatment recommendations provided by your healthcare professional. Treatment options vary depending on the specific sleep disorder but may include behavioral therapies, medication, continuous positive airway pressure (CPAP) therapy, or lifestyle changes.

**4. Establish a Consistent Sleep Schedule:** Maintain a regular sleep schedule by going to bed and waking up at the same time every day, even on weekends. This helps regulate your body's internal clock and improves sleep quality.

**5. Create a Relaxing Bedtime Routine:** Develop a calming bedtime routine to signal your body that it's time to wind down. This could include activities like

reading, gentle stretching, or practicing relaxation techniques like Progressive Muscle Relaxation (PMR) or meditation.

**6. Optimize Your Sleep Environment:** Make your bedroom conducive to sleep by keeping it dark, quiet, and at a comfortable temperature. Consider using blackout curtains, earplugs, or a white noise machine to block out disturbances.

**7. Limit Screen Time Before Bed:** Minimize exposure to screens (phones, computers, TVs) at least an hour before bedtime. The blue light from screens can disrupt the production of the sleep hormone melatonin.

**8. Manage Stress and Anxiety:** Practice stress-reduction techniques such as deep breathing, meditation, or yoga throughout the day to ease your mind before bedtime.

**9. Limit Caffeine and Stimulants:** Reduce or eliminate the consumption of caffeine and other stimulants, especially in the afternoon and evening.

**10. Avoid Heavy Meals and Alcohol Before Bed:** Avoid heavy meals close to bedtime and limit alcohol intake, as both can disrupt sleep patterns.

**11. Stay Active During the Day:** Engage in regular physical activity during the day, as exercise can help improve sleep quality. However, avoid vigorous exercise close to bedtime.

**12. Monitor Your Sleep:** Keep a sleep diary to track your sleep patterns and any factors that may affect your sleep. This can help you identify patterns and make necessary adjustments.

**13. Be Patient and Persistent:** Overcoming sleep disorders may take time and consistent effort. Be patient with yourself and stay committed to implementing healthy sleep habits.

If your sleep disorder persists despite making lifestyle changes, or if it significantly affects your quality of life, consult with your healthcare professional to explore other treatment options or interventions. Remember that with the right approach and support, many people successfully manage and overcome sleep disorders, leading to improved overall well-being and vitality.

## *Identifying Common Sleep Disorders Affecting The Target Age Group*

Sleep disorders can affect individuals of all ages, including children, adolescents, adults, and the elderly. While some sleep disorders can occur at any age, certain disorders are more prevalent within specific age groups. Here are some common sleep disorders affecting different age groups:

**1. Infants and Children:**

- Sleep-Onset Association Disorder: Difficulty falling asleep without specific sleep associations (e.g., rocking, nursing, or being held).

- Night Wakings or Night Terrors: Frequent awakenings during the night or episodes of sudden awakening accompanied by intense fear or agitation.

- Sleep-Related Breathing Disorders: Conditions like sleep apnea, are characterized by pauses in breathing during sleep.

**2. Adolescents and Young Adults:**

- Delayed Sleep Phase Syndrome: A tendency to stay awake and fall asleep later at night, leading to difficulty waking up in the morning.

- Insomnia: Difficulty falling asleep or staying asleep, often due to stress, anxiety, or lifestyle factors.

- Restless Legs Syndrome (RLS): An urge to move the legs, often accompanied by discomfort, that worsens in the evening or at night.

**3. Adults:**

- Insomnia: Persistent difficulty falling asleep or staying

asleep, which can be caused by various factors, including stress, anxiety, and medical conditions.

- Sleep Apnea: A sleep-related breathing disorder characterized by repeated interruptions in breathing during sleep.

- Narcolepsy: A neurological disorder causing excessive daytime sleepiness and sudden episodes of sleep attacks.

**4. Elderly Adults:**

- Sleep Apnea: The prevalence of sleep apnea increases with age, particularly in older adults with other health conditions.

- Periodic Limb Movement Disorder (PLMD): Involuntary leg movements during sleep, which can cause sleep disruption.

- Insomnia: Occurs more frequently in the elderly due to various factors, including changes in sleep patterns and health conditions.

It's important to note that these are general trends and individuals within each age group may experience sleep disorders differently. The prevalence and severity of sleep disorders can also vary depending on individual factors, such as lifestyle, genetics, and underlying health conditions. If you or someone you know is experiencing significant sleep disturbances, it is essential to seek a proper evaluation and diagnosis from a healthcare professional or a sleep specialist. Early identification and appropriate management of sleep disorders can lead to improved sleep quality and overall well-being.

## Seeking Professional Help And Resources For Sleep-Related Issues

If you are experiencing sleep-related issues, seeking professional help is essential to identify the underlying causes and receive appropriate treatment. Here are some resources and professionals you can reach out to for assistance:

- **Primary Care Physician:** Start by scheduling an appointment with your primary care physician. They can conduct an initial evaluation, discuss your sleep concerns, and may refer you to a sleep specialist if necessary.

- **Sleep Specialist:** If your sleep issues require further investigation or specialized care, a sleep specialist is a medical professional with expertise in sleep disorders. They can perform comprehensive evaluations, order sleep studies (polysomnography), and provide tailored treatment plans.

- **Sleep Clinics and Centers:** Sleep clinics and centers are specialized facilities that focus on diagnosing and treating various sleep disorders. They offer comprehensive evaluations, sleep studies, and access to a team of experts in sleep medicine.

- **Therapists and Counselors:** For sleep issues related to stress, anxiety, or emotional concerns, mental health professionals, such as therapists and counselors, can provide support through cognitive-behavioral therapy for insomnia (CBT-I) or other therapeutic techniques.

- **Online Sleep Resources:** There are numerous reputable online resources dedicated to sleep health. Websites from sleep organizations, sleep clinics, and medical associations often provide valuable information, sleep tips, and self-assessment tools.

- **Sleep Apps:** There are several smartphone apps designed to track sleep patterns, provide relaxation exercises, and offer sleep-related tips. Some apps may also offer CBT-I programs.

- **Books and Publications:** Look for books and publications authored by sleep experts that cover various sleep disorders and effective strategies for improving sleep.

- **Sleep Support Groups:** Local or online sleep support groups can connect you with individuals facing similar sleep-related challenges. Sharing experiences and strategies with others can be beneficial.

- **Sleep Wellness Programs:** Some wellness centers or community organizations offer sleep-related workshops or programs that focus on healthy sleep habits and stress reduction techniques.

**When seeking professional help or utilizing resources, remember to:**

- Be open and honest about your sleep concerns and any other relevant health issues.

- Share information about your sleep patterns, lifestyle, and daily routines.

- Discuss any medications or supplements you are taking, as they may impact sleep.

- Ask questions and seek clarification about any recommendations or treatments offered.

Addressing sleep-related issues is important for your overall well-being. Don't hesitate to seek help, as many sleep disorders are treatable, and improving your sleep quality can have a positive impact on various aspects of your life.

## *Lifestyle Changes And Techniques To Manage Specific Sleep Disorders*

Managing specific sleep disorders often involves a combination of lifestyle changes and specific techniques tailored to each disorder. Here are some lifestyle changes and techniques that can help manage common sleep disorders:

**1. Insomnia:**

- Maintain a consistent sleep schedule: Go to bed and wake up at the same time every day, even on weekends.

- Create a relaxing bedtime routine: Engage in calming activities like reading, taking a warm bath, or practicing relaxation techniques.

- Limit caffeine and alcohol: Avoid consuming caffeine and alcohol close to bedtime, as they can disrupt sleep.

- Manage stress: Practice stress-reduction techniques such as deep breathing, meditation, or yoga during the day to ease your mind before bedtime.

- Limit screen time: Minimize exposure to screens (phones, computers, TVs) at least an hour before bedtime to avoid disruptions to your sleep-wake cycle.

**2. Sleep Apnea:**

- Maintain a healthy weight: Losing weight if overweight can help reduce sleep apnea symptoms.

- Sleep on your side: Sleeping on your side may reduce the severity of sleep apnea compared to sleeping on your back.

- Elevate your head: Using a wedge pillow or adjustable bed to elevate your head can improve breathing during sleep.

- Avoid alcohol and sedatives: These substances can relax the muscles in the throat and worsen sleep apnea.

## 3. Restless Legs Syndrome (RLS):

- Identify triggers: Keep a diary to identify triggers that worsen RLS symptoms, such as certain foods or medications.

- Regular exercise: Engage in regular, moderate exercise, but avoid vigorous exercise close to bedtime.

- Warm baths or massages: Soaking in a warm bath or receiving a gentle massage before bedtime can help relax the legs.

## 4. Narcolepsy:

- Schedule short naps: Short daytime naps (15-20 minutes) can help manage excessive sleepiness in narcolepsy.

- Stimulants: Medications like modafinil or amphetamines can help improve wakefulness in narcolepsy.

## 5. Delayed Sleep Phase Syndrome:

- Gradual sleep schedule adjustments: Gradually shift your bedtime and wake-up time earlier each day until you reach your desired schedule.

- Morning sunlight exposure: Get natural sunlight exposure in the morning to help regulate your internal clock.

## 6. Sleep-Related Breathing Disorders (e.g., sleepwalking, night terrors):

- Create a safe sleep environment: Remove any obstacles or hazards from the sleeping area to prevent injury during sleepwalking episodes.

- Relaxation techniques: Practice relaxation exercises or mindfulness before bedtime to reduce the likelihood of night terrors.

It's important to note that these recommendations are general guidelines and may not apply to every individual with a specific sleep disorder. For personalized advice and treatment, it's best to consult with a healthcare professional or a sleep specialist. They can provide tailored strategies and, if needed, recommend specific treatments or therapies to manage your specific sleep disorder effectively.

# CHAPTER 11: MAINTAINING A CONSISTENT SLEEP SCHEDULE

Maintaining a consistent sleep schedule is crucial for improving sleep quality and overall well-being. Our bodies have a natural internal clock, known as the circadian rhythm, which regulates our sleep-wake cycle. Consistency in sleep timing helps synchronize this internal clock, making it easier to fall asleep, stay asleep, and wake up feeling refreshed. Here are some tips to help you establish and maintain a consistent sleep schedule:

**1. Set a Fixed Bedtime and Wake-Up Time:** Determine the time you need to wake up each morning and calculate the number of hours of sleep you need. Set a bedtime that allows you to get the recommended amount of sleep for your age group (typically 7-9 hours for adults).

**2. Stick to the Same Schedule Every Day:** Try to maintain the same sleep schedule, even on weekends and holidays. Consistency is essential for regulating your circadian rhythm.

**3. Gradually Adjust Your Sleep Schedule:** If you need to make significant changes to your sleep schedule (e.g., due to shift work or travel), do it gradually. Gradually adjust your bedtime and wake-up time by 15-30 minutes each day until you reach your desired schedule.

**4. Avoid Sleeping In:** As tempting as it may be to catch up on sleep on weekends, avoid sleeping in excessively. Oversleeping can disrupt your circadian rhythm and make it harder to fall asleep at the desired time the following night.

**5. Create a Relaxing Bedtime Routine:** Establish a calming bedtime routine that signals your body it's time to wind down. This may include activities like reading, taking a warm bath, practicing relaxation techniques, or listening to soothing music.

**6. Limit Stimulants and Heavy Meals:** Avoid consuming caffeine, nicotine, and heavy meals close to bedtime, as they can interfere with sleep quality.

**7. Get Sunlight Exposure in the Morning:** Exposure to natural sunlight in the morning helps regulate your circadian rhythm. Spend time outdoors or open your curtains to let in natural light soon after waking up.

**8. Limit Bright Lights in the Evening:** Minimize exposure to bright lights, especially from electronic devices, in the evening before bedtime. The blue light emitted by screens can interfere with melatonin production, making it harder to fall asleep.

**9. Create a Sleep-Conducive Environment:** Make your bedroom a comfortable and sleep-friendly environment. Keep the room cool, dark, and quiet, and invest in a comfortable mattress and pillows.

**10. Be Patient and Persistent:** It may take a few weeks to adjust to a new sleep schedule and experience the full benefits of a consistent sleep routine. Be patient and persistent in maintaining your schedule.

By maintaining a consistent sleep schedule, you can improve your sleep quality, increase daytime energy levels, and support overall health and well-being. Remember that everyone's sleep needs are different, so pay attention to how you feel during the day to determine if you are getting enough restful sleep. If you consistently have difficulty sleeping or feel excessively tired during the day, consider consulting a healthcare professional or a sleep specialist for further evaluation and guidance.

## The Importance Of Regular Sleep-Wake Cycles For Quality Rest

Regular sleep-wake cycles, also known as consistent sleep schedules, are vital for achieving quality rest and maintaining overall health and well-being. Here are some key reasons why regular sleep-wake cycles are essential:

**1. Synchronization of Circadian Rhythm:** Our bodies have an internal biological clock, known as the circadian rhythm, which regulates the timing of various physiological processes, including sleep. Consistency in sleep timing helps synchronize this internal clock, making it easier to fall asleep and wake up at the desired times.

**2. Improved Sleep Quality:** Regular sleep schedules lead to better sleep quality. When you go to bed and wake up at the same time each day, your body is better prepared to enter the different stages of sleep more efficiently. This allows you to experience more deep sleep and REM sleep, which are crucial for physical and mental restoration.

**3. Enhanced Daytime Alertness:** By maintaining consistent sleep-wake cycles, you can establish a steady sleep routine that optimizes your alertness and productivity during the day. This, in turn, can improve cognitive function, concentration, and overall performance.

**4. Balanced Hormone Production:** Sleep is essential for hormone regulation, including those involved in appetite (ghrelin and leptin) and stress (cortisol). Irregular sleep schedules can disrupt hormone production, potentially leading to imbalances and health issues.

**5. Improved Mood and Emotional Well-being:** Consistent sleep schedules contribute to emotional stability and overall well-being. Sudden changes in sleep patterns can negatively impact mood and increase the risk of mood disorders like depression and anxiety.

**6. Better Sleep Onset and Maintenance:** Going to bed at the same time each night helps signal to your body that it's time to sleep. This reduces the time it takes to fall asleep (sleep latency) and improves your ability to stay asleep throughout the night.

**7. Enhanced Sleep Efficiency:** Sleep efficiency refers to the percentage of time spent asleep while in bed. Consistent sleep-wake cycles increase sleep efficiency, allowing you to spend more time asleep relative to the time spent in bed.

**8. Strengthened Immune System:** Adequate and consistent sleep supports a robust immune system, making you more resilient to illnesses and infections.

**9. Reduced Risk of Sleep Disorders:** Regular sleep schedules can help prevent the development of certain sleep disorders, such as insomnia, circadian rhythm disorders, and shift work sleep disorders.

**10. Overall Health Benefits:** Good sleep hygiene, which includes regular sleep-wake cycles, is associated with numerous health benefits, such as better cardiovascular health, improved metabolism, and a reduced risk of chronic health conditions.

In conclusion, maintaining regular sleep-wake cycles is essential for promoting quality rest, overall health, and optimal functioning during the day. Consistency in sleep schedules helps regulate the internal body clock, enhances sleep quality, and supports various physiological and psychological processes critical for well-being. Prioritize getting enough sleep and adhering to a consistent sleep routine to reap the many benefits of restful and restorative sleep.

## *Strategies For Establishing And Maintaining A Consistent Sleep Schedule*

Establishing and maintaining a consistent sleep schedule requires commitment and a few strategies to help regulate your circadian rhythm and promote better sleep. Here are some effective strategies to help you establish and maintain a consistent sleep schedule:

**1. Set a Regular Bedtime and Wake-Up Time:**

- Determine the ideal amount of sleep you need based on your age and lifestyle, and set a consistent bedtime and wake-up time every day, including weekends.

- Aim for 7-9 hours of sleep per night for most adults.

**2. Gradually Adjust Your Sleep Schedule:**

- If you need to shift your sleep schedule, do it gradually. Adjust your bedtime and wake-up time by 15-30 minutes each day until you reach your desired schedule.

- Allow your body time to adapt to the changes in your sleep routine.

**3. Create a Relaxing Bedtime Routine:**

- Establish a calming pre-sleep routine to signal your body that it's time to wind down. This may include activities like reading a book, taking a warm bath, or practicing relaxation techniques.

- Try to avoid stimulating activities, bright screens, and intense discussions right before bedtime.

## 4. Limit Napping:

- If you have trouble falling asleep at night, avoid long or late-afternoon naps, as they can interfere with your ability to sleep at bedtime.

- If you need to nap during the day, keep it short (20-30 minutes) and earlier in the day.

## 5. Create a Sleep-Conducive Environment:

- Make your bedroom comfortable and conducive to sleep. Keep the room dark, quiet, and at a comfortable temperature.

- Invest in a supportive mattress and pillows to improve sleep quality.

## 6. Practice Consistent Meal Times:

- Maintain regular meal times, and avoid heavy or spicy meals close to bedtime, as they can disrupt sleep.

- If you need a snack before bedtime, choose something light and easily digestible.

## 7. Limit Caffeine and Stimulants:

- Avoid consuming caffeine or other stimulants close to bedtime, as they can interfere with your ability to fall asleep.

- Be mindful of hidden sources of caffeine, such as certain medications and energy drinks.

## 8. Get Sunlight Exposure During the Day:

- Exposure to natural sunlight during the day helps regulate your circadian rhythm. Spend time outdoors or near windows to receive sunlight exposure.

## 9. Stay Active During the Day:

- Engage in regular physical activity during the day, as it can promote better sleep at night.

- However, avoid vigorous exercise close to bedtime, as it may make it harder to fall asleep.

**10. Be Consistent Even on Weekends:**

- Try to maintain your sleep schedule, even on weekends and holidays, to support your body's natural sleep-wake cycle.

**11. Monitor Your Sleep:** Keep a sleep diary to track your sleep patterns and any factors that may affect your sleep. This can help you identify patterns and make necessary adjustments.

Remember that establishing a consistent sleep schedule may take some time and patience. Stick to your routine and make adjustments as needed to find what works best for you. If you continue to have difficulty maintaining a consistent sleep schedule or experience persistent sleep issues, consider consulting a healthcare professional or a sleep specialist for further evaluation and guidance.

## Coping With Disruptions
## And Managing Jet Lag

Coping with disruptions to your sleep schedule and managing jet lag can be challenging, but with the right strategies, you can minimize the impact on your sleep and help your body adjust more quickly. Here are some tips to help you cope with disruptions and manage jet lag effectively:

**1. Gradual Time Adjustments:** If you know you'll be facing a significant time zone change, start adjusting your sleep schedule gradually a few days before your trip. Go to bed and wake up 15-30 minutes earlier or later each day, depending on the direction of travel.

**2. Stay Hydrated:** Drink plenty of water before, during, and after your travel to stay hydrated. Avoid excessive caffeine and alcohol, as they can disrupt your sleep.

**3. Get Sunlight Exposure:** Upon arrival at your destination, spend time outdoors and expose yourself to natural sunlight. Sunlight helps regulate your circadian rhythm and helps your body adapt to the new time zone.

**4. Nap Strategically:** If you're feeling extremely tired upon arrival, take a short nap (20-30 minutes) to help you stay alert. Avoid long naps or napping too close to bedtime, as it can interfere with your ability to sleep at night.

**5. Use Sleep Aids Sparingly:** While it may be tempting to use sleep aids, such as medication or supplements, to help you sleep during travel or adjust to a new time zone, use them sparingly and only under the guidance of a healthcare professional.

**6. Stay Active:** Engage in light physical activity, such as walking, stretching, or gentle exercises, to help reduce fatigue and promote better sleep.

**7. Practice Good Sleep Hygiene:** Stick to your regular bedtime routine and practice good sleep hygiene at your destination. Keep the sleep environment dark, quiet, and comfortable to support restful sleep.

**8. Avoid Heavy Meals and Stimulants:** Avoid heavy meals close to bedtime, and limit caffeine and other stimulants in the evening, as they can disrupt your ability to fall asleep.

**9. Stay Patient and Give Yourself Time:** It can take a few days for your body to fully adjust to a new time zone. Be patient with yourself and give your body time to acclimate.

**10. Choose Flights Wisely:** If possible, choose flights that arrive at your destination in the early evening to help you stay awake until bedtime. Avoid arriving late at night, as it may be more challenging to adjust to a new sleep schedule.

**11. Use Sleep-Enhancing Apps:** Some smartphone apps offer relaxation exercises, white noise, or guided meditations that can help you relax and sleep better during travel or in unfamiliar environments.

Remember that each person's ability to cope with disruptions and manage jet lag may vary. It's essential to find what works best for you. If jet lag or sleep disruptions persist for an extended period, consult a healthcare professional or a sleep specialist for further guidance and support.

# CHAPTER 12: EMBRACING A SLEEP-ENHANCING LIFESTYLE

Embracing a sleep-enhancing lifestyle involves adopting habits and practices that prioritize and support healthy sleep. By making positive changes to your daily routine and sleep environment, you can improve the quality and duration of your sleep. Here are some tips for embracing a sleep-enhancing lifestyle:

**1. Stick to a Consistent Sleep Schedule:** Go to bed and wake up at the same time every day, even on weekends. Consistency helps regulate your circadian rhythm and improves sleep quality.

**2. Create a Relaxing Bedtime Routine:** Develop a calming pre-sleep routine to signal your body that it's time to wind down. This may include activities like reading, taking a warm bath, or practicing relaxation techniques.

**3. Limit Caffeine and Stimulants:** Avoid consuming caffeine and other stimulants close to bedtime, as they can disrupt sleep.

**4. Avoid Heavy Meals Before Bedtime:** Limit heavy or spicy meals close to bedtime, as they can cause discomfort and disrupt sleep.

**5. Create a Comfortable Sleep Environment:** Make your bedroom a sleep-conducive environment. Keep the room dark, quiet, and at a comfortable temperature. Invest in a supportive mattress and pillows.

**6. Limit Screen Time Before Bed:** Minimize exposure to screens (phones, computers, TVs) at least an hour before bedtime. The blue light from screens can interfere with melatonin production, making it harder to fall asleep.

**7. Get Regular Exercise:** Engage in regular physical activity, as it can promote better sleep. Aim for at least 30 minutes of moderate exercise most days of the week, but avoid vigorous exercise close to bedtime.

**8. Manage Stress and Anxiety:** Practice stress-reduction techniques such as deep breathing, meditation, or yoga throughout the day to ease your mind before bedtime.

**9. Limit Daytime Napping:** Keep daytime naps short (20-30 minutes) and earlier in the day to avoid interfering with nighttime sleep.

**10. Limit Alcohol Intake:** While alcohol may initially make you feel drowsy, it can disrupt sleep patterns and lead to fragmented sleep.

**11. Monitor Your Sleep:** Keep a sleep diary to track your sleep patterns and any factors that may affect your sleep. This can help you identify patterns and make necessary adjustments.

**12. Seek Natural Sunlight Exposure:** Get exposure to natural sunlight during the day, especially in the morning, to help regulate your circadian rhythm.

**13. Avoid Clock Watching:** If you wake up during the night, try to avoid checking the clock. Constantly looking at the time can increase anxiety and make it harder to fall back asleep.

By incorporating these sleep-enhancing practices into your daily life, you can create a healthy sleep routine that supports restful and restorative sleep. Prioritize your sleep, and remember that small changes in your lifestyle can make a significant difference in your sleep quality and overall well-being. If you continue to have sleep difficulties, consider consulting a healthcare professional or a sleep specialist for further evaluation and personalized guidance.

## Summarizing Key Techniques From The Book To Improve Sleep Quality

The book outlines various techniques to improve sleep quality. Here is a summary of some key techniques:

- **Consistent Sleep Schedule:** Maintain a regular sleep-wake schedule by going to bed and waking up at the same time every day, even on weekends.

- **Bedtime Routine:** Establish a calming bedtime routine to signal your body that it's time to wind down. This may include activities like reading, taking a warm bath, or practicing relaxation techniques.

- **Sleep-Conducive Environment:** Make your bedroom comfortable and conducive to sleep by keeping it dark, quiet, and at a comfortable temperature. Invest in a supportive mattress and pillows.

- **Limit Screen Time Before Bed:** Minimize exposure to screens (phones, computers, TVs) at least an hour before bedtime to avoid disruptions to your sleep-wake cycle caused by blue light.

- **Mindfulness and Relaxation Techniques:** Practice mindfulness, deep breathing, meditation, or yoga to manage stress and anxiety before bedtime.

- **Limit Caffeine and Stimulants:** Avoid consuming caffeine and other stimulants close to bedtime, as they can interfere with your ability to fall asleep.

- **Regular Exercise:** Engage in regular physical activity during the day, but avoid vigorous exercise close to bedtime.

- **Monitor Sleep Patterns:** Keep a sleep diary to track your sleep patterns and identify factors that may affect your sleep.

- **Natural Sunlight Exposure:** Get exposure to natural sunlight during the day, especially in the morning, to help regulate your circadian rhythm.

- **Limit Daytime Napping:** Keep daytime naps short (20-30 minutes) and earlier in the day to avoid interfering with nighttime sleep.

- **Avoid Heavy Meals and Alcohol Before Bed:** Avoid heavy or spicy meals close to bedtime and limit alcohol intake, as both can disrupt sleep patterns.

- **Stress Management:** Practice stress-reduction techniques throughout the day to ease your mind before bedtime.

- **Seek Professional Help:** If you continue to experience sleep difficulties, consider consulting a healthcare professional or a sleep specialist for further evaluation and personalized guidance.

By incorporating these techniques into your daily life, you can create a sleep-enhancing lifestyle that promotes restful and restorative sleep. Remember that everyone's sleep needs are different, so find what works best for you and prioritize your sleep to improve overall well-being.

## Encouraging Long-Term Lifestyle Changes For Lasting Results

Encouraging long-term lifestyle changes is essential for achieving lasting results in improving sleep quality and overall well-being. Here are some strategies to promote sustainable changes:

**1. Gradual Implementation:** Introduce lifestyle changes gradually rather than trying to overhaul your entire routine all at once. Focus on one or two changes at a time, allowing yourself to adjust and form new habits.

**2. Set Realistic Goals:** Set achievable and realistic goals for yourself. Be patient with the process, as lasting changes take time and consistency.

**3. Consistency is Key:** Stick to your new sleep-enhancing habits consistently. The more you practice them, the more they become ingrained in your daily routine.

**4. Create a Supportive Environment:** Surround yourself with supportive individuals who encourage and understand your efforts to improve sleep.

**5. Celebrate Progress:** Acknowledge and celebrate your progress, no matter how small. Celebrating milestones can motivate you to continue making positive changes.

**6. Self-Compassion:** Be kind to yourself throughout the process. Recognize that setbacks are a normal part of change and view them as opportunities to learn and grow.

**7. Build a Strong Foundation:** Focus on building a strong foundation for good sleep hygiene, such as maintaining a consistent sleep schedule and creating a sleep-conducive environment.

**8. Engage in Mindful Eating:** Pay attention to your eating habits and make conscious choices about what you consume. A balanced diet can positively impact sleep.

**9. Stay Active:** Continue engaging in regular physical activity that you enjoy. Physical exercise supports healthy sleep and overall well-being.

**10. Manage Stress Effectively:** Develop stress-reduction techniques, such as mindfulness, meditation, or relaxation exercises, to manage stress and promote better sleep.

**11. Be Patient and Persistent:** Lasting lifestyle changes take time. Be patient with yourself, and stay persistent in your efforts to improve sleep quality.

**12. Continuously Learn and Adapt:** Stay informed about the latest sleep research and sleep improvement strategies. Adapt your approach as needed based on what works best for you.

**13. Prioritize Sleep as a Health Goal:** View sleep as a vital component of your overall health and well-being. Recognize the importance of good sleep for your physical, mental, and emotional health.

By focusing on lasting lifestyle changes, you can create a sustainable foundation for better sleep and improved overall health. It's not about quick fixes but rather adopting habits and behaviors that become an integral part of your daily life. Remember that small, consistent steps can lead to significant improvements in your sleep quality and overall quality of life.

## *Celebrating Improved Sleep And Its Positive Impact On Overall Well-Being*

Celebrating improved sleep and recognizing its positive impact on overall well-being is an important part of the journey to better health and happiness. Improved sleep can have far-reaching effects on various aspects of our lives, and taking the time to acknowledge these benefits can be motivating and encouraging. Here are some reasons to celebrate improved sleep and its positive impact:

1. **Enhanced Energy and Vitality:** With better sleep, you wake up feeling more refreshed and energized, ready to tackle the day's challenges with enthusiasm.

2. **Improved Mood and Emotional Well-being:** Quality sleep is closely linked to emotional stability and mental well-being. Improved sleep can lead to a more positive outlook on life and better emotional resilience.

3. **Enhanced Cognitive Functioning:** When you get enough restful sleep, your brain functions at its best. Improved focus, concentration, and memory recall are among the cognitive benefits of quality sleep.

4. **Increased Productivity and Performance:** Better sleep allows you to be more productive and efficient in your daily tasks, both at work and in your personal life.

5. **Strengthened Immune System:** Adequate sleep plays a critical role in supporting a healthy immune system, making you more resilient to illnesses and infections.

6. **Better Physical Health:** Improved sleep is associated with better cardiovascular health, a balanced metabolism, and a reduced risk of chronic health conditions.

7. **Stress Reduction:** Quality sleep can significantly reduce stress

levels and help you manage life's challenges with greater ease.

**8. Enhanced Creativity and Problem-Solving Abilities:** Restful sleep fosters creativity and enhances your ability to come up with innovative solutions to problems.

**9. Positive Impact on Relationships:** Improved sleep can lead to a more positive and harmonious atmosphere in relationships, as adequate rest supports better communication and emotional regulation.

**10. Overall Sense of Well-Being:** When you prioritize sleep and experience its positive effects, you may notice an overall improvement in your sense of well-being and happiness.

**11. Personal Growth and Self-Care:** Making sleep a priority is a form of self-care and demonstrates your commitment to taking care of your physical and mental health.

**12. Inspiring Others:** Your dedication to improving sleep and reaping its benefits can inspire others to prioritize their sleep health.

By recognizing and celebrating these positive impacts, you reinforce the importance of sleep as a fundamental pillar of overall well-being. Take the time to appreciate the progress you've made, and use the positive outcomes as motivation to continue prioritizing sleep and embracing a sleep-enhancing lifestyle. Remember that improved sleep is a valuable investment in your health and happiness, and it's worth celebrating every step of the way.